# HOW TO COPE WITH ANAEMIA

DR JOAN GOMEZ is Honorary Consulting Psychiatrist to the Chelsea and Westminster Hospital. She was trained at King's College, London, and Westminster Hospital, qualifying MB, BS, and obtained her DPM and MRCPsych in 1973 and 1974 respectively. She was elected a Fellow of the Royal College of Psychiatrists in 1982, and obtained the Diploma in the History of Medicine in 1996. She is a Fellow of the Society of Apothecaries and also of the Royal Society of Medicine. She has been engaged in clinical work and research on the interface between psychiatry and physical medicine. Dr Gomez is also the author of three other books published by Sheldon Press: *Coping with Thyroid Problems* (1994), *How to Cope with Bulimia* (1995) and *Living with Diabetes* (1995). Her husband was a general practitioner and they have ten children.

GW00357792

# Overcoming Common Problems Series

For a full list of titles please contact
Sheldon Press, Marylebone Road, London NW1 4DU

**The Assertiveness Workbook**
A plan for busy women
JOANNA GUTMANN

**Birth Over Thirty Five**
SHEILA KITZINGER

**Body Language**
How to read others' thoughts by their
gestures
ALLAN PEASE

**Body Language in Relationships**
DAVID COHEN

**Cancer – A Family Affair**
NEVILLE SHONE

**Coping Successfully with Hayfever**
DR ROBERT YOUNGSON

**Coping Successfully with Migraine**
SUE DYSON

**Coping Successfully with Pain**
NEVILLE SHONE

**Coping Successfully with Your Irritable
Bowel**
ROSEMARY NICOL

**Coping with Anxiety and Depression**
SHIRLEY TRICKETT

**Coping with Breast Cancer**
DR EADIE HEYDERMAN

**Coping with Bronchitis and Emphysema**
DR TOM SMITH

**Coping with Chronic Fatigue**
TRUDIE CHALDER

**Coping with Depression and Elation**
DR PATRICK McKEON

**Curing Arthritis Diet Book**
MARGARET HILLS

**Curing Arthritis – The Drug-Free Way**
MARGARET HILLS

**Depression**
DR PAUL HAUCK

**Divorce and Separation**
Every woman's guide to a new life
ANGELA WILLANS

**Everything Parents Should Know About
Drugs**
SARAH LAWSON

**Good Stress Guide, The**
MARY HARTLEY

**Heart Attacks – Prevent and Survive**
DR TOM SMITH

**Helping Children Cope with Grief**
ROSEMARY WELLS

**How to Improve Your Confidence**
DR KENNETH HAMBLY

**How to Interview and Be Interviewed**
MICHELE BROWN AND GYLES
BRANDRETH

**How to Keep Your Cholesterol in Check**
DR ROBERT POVEY

**How to Pass Your Driving Test**
DONALD RIDLAND

**How to Start a Conversation and Make
Friends**
DON GABOR

**How to Write a Successful CV**
JOANNA GUTMANN

**Hysterectomy**
SUZIE HAYMAN

**The Irritable Bowel Diet Book**
ROSEMARY NICOL

**Overcoming Guilt**
DR WINDY DRYDEN

**The Parkinson's Disease Handbook**
DR RICHARD GODWIN-AUSTEN

**Talking About Anorexia**
How to cope with life without starving
MAROUSHKA MONRO

**Think Your Way to Happiness**
DR WINDY DRYDEN AND JACK
GORDON

**Overcoming Common Problems**

# How to Cope with Anaemia

Dr Joan Gomez

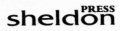

First published in Great Britain in 1998 by
Sheldon Press, SPCK, Marylebone Road, London NW1 4DU

British Library Cataloguing-in-Publication Data
A catalogue for this book is available from the British Library

ISBN 0–85969–788–6


Photoset by Deltatype Limited, Birkenhead, Merseyside
Printed in Great Britain by
Biddles Ltd, Guildford and King's Lynn

# Contents

To Sharon, with love

# 1
## What is anaemia?

Anaemia isn't fashionable – you don't hear people boasting that they've had it or health freaks extolling the virtues of some wonderful new treatment for it. To be honest, 'anaemia' has a Dickensian ring. In fact, the word came into use in England around 1836, shortly before Queen Victoria came to the throne. The Victorians took anaemia seriously, and the drug manufacturers of the time made their fortunes with Pink Pills for Pale People, Iron Jelloids and the like. Nowadays, although we don't talk about it very much, anaemia hasn't gone away; it is very common and causes a great deal of 'subhealth' as well as more serious illnesses.

Anaemia – Greek for 'no blood' – means, in practice, a shortage of haemoglobin. This vital molecule – half protein, half pigment – colours your blood red and transports vital oxygen to every single one of the 75 trillion cells in your body. Anaemia isn't an illness in itself, like measles or arthritis, but is always the result of something else going wrong. The underlying disorder may be a deficiency of iron or the particular vitamins needed for making haemoglobin, leaking away of blood from an ulcer or a pile, thyroid deficiency, certain poisons . . . or one of many other unrelated problems. So, if your doctor discovers that you are anaemic, this is the beginning of a detective trail to find out why. Only then can the right treatment begin.

### *What is so special about haemoglobin that it matters so much?*

'Haem' is the red colouring, 'globin' the protein part. Joined together, they make a molecule that has the unique quality of being able to grab onto a supply of oxygen as it is swept along in the blood through your lungs. In fact, haemogoblin enables your blood to carry 50 times as much oxygen as it could take otherwise. And it is oxygen that makes your blood truly lifeblood.

When it reaches the tissues, the haemoglobin lets go of just as much oxygen as that particular tissue needs at that particular time. For instance, when you are taking vigorous exercise, the haemoglobin gives up much more of its oxygen, and it adjusts the amount automatically when you climb a mountain or reach a high altitude in a plane. Also, when the haemoglobin arrives in the tissues, it is 97 per cent saturated with oxygen and it is bright pillar-box red. There the oxygen is used in the slow combustion process of the various nutrients in the blood, such as sugar and fat, and is converted into carbon dioxide. This, in turn, is picked up by the blood, which then becomes a dark cherry red, and carried back through the lungs where you can breathe it out. There, more oxygen is taken on board by the haemoglobin and the cycle begins again. This continuous process is the essence of life – for every cell in your body.

As haemoglobin is so remarkable and precious, it doesn't just wash around in the fluid part of your blood with the food products, hormones and various other chemicals, but travels in special, flexible containers: the red blood corpuscles. One way of assessing how much haemoglobin you have is by counting the number of red cells: a blood count. They are the most numerous cells in your body – you have millions upon millions. Men have about 5 per cent more than women, with the equivalent extra haemoglobin, and how many you have also varies with age, as shown in Table 1.1.

Table 1.1   Variations in blood counts

| Sectors of the population | Blood counts |
|---|---|
| Men | 4.5–6.5 million per cubic mm |
| Women | 3.8–5.8 million per cubic mm |
| A newborn baby | 4 million per cubic mm on average |
| A three-month-old baby | 3.2 million per cubic mm |
| A one-year-old child | 3.6 million per cubic mm |
| A ten-year-old child | 4.2 million per cubic mm |

Apart from the differences due to sex and age, the number of red cells in the blood varies naturally during the course of a day, when you have a meal, a drink or take exercise. It increases when you feel strong emotion – especially anger, fear or simply excitement. Physical stress, lack of oxygen in the air, a cold shower or someone massaging – or tickling – your abdomen can also have the same effect. The increase is brought about by your body calling on your reserves, which are in your spleen (located under your lower ribs on the left side of your body). The aim of this is to increase the amount of haemoglobin in circulation so as to maximize the amount of oxygen carried to the tissues.

A low count of red cells spells anaemia. There may have been a fault in the manufacturing process or an undue loss of the cells.

There are two kinds of human haemoglobin: haemoglobin F and haemoglobin A. 'F' stands for foetal or immature, 'A' for adult. Thus an unborn baby has type F, and a young child a mixture of types A and F. Adults have almost all type A. During pregnancy, mothers-to-be have about 25 per cent of the F kind in their blood, because that is what their babies need.

As you would expect, the number of red blood cells relates directly to the amount of haemoglobin in your blood, so there are the same sex and age differences as before (see Table 1.2).

Table 1.2   Haemoglobin concentration in the blood

| Sex and age groups | Grams per 1ml of blood |
|---|---|
| Men | 13.6–18 |
| Women | 11.5–16.4 |
| A newborn baby | 13.6–19.6 |
| A three-month-old baby | 9.5–12.5 (milk alone does not provide all the ingredients to make blood) |
| A one-year-old child | 11–13 (on a mixed diet) |
| A ten-year-old child | 11.5–14.8 |
| Elderly men | 13.62 (on average) |
| Elderly women | 13.11 |

You can see from Table 1.2 which are the two dangerous times for anaemia – they are at the extremes of life. For women there is another important time – during pregnancy. These three anaemia-prone periods are physiologically based, not the result of an illness but a perfectly natural part of life. Nevertheless, these are times when we should take extra care, for instance with diet and avoiding excessive exercise, which, as we have seen, puts a strain on our haemoglobin resources. Most women know they need adequate iron during pregnancy, but not many men or women take the same trouble when they reach retirement age.

## Why does a shortage of haemoglobin matter?

Clearly, when you are pregnant and your baby is growing and developing at a phenomenal rate, the progress the baby makes will be impeded if it is deprived of a supply of first-class blood from you. The size, strength and, above all, the long-term mental development of the baby may suffer. You share your blood with the baby and it is not until after three months into the pregnancy that the baby begins to make blood for itself. In any case, all the raw materials are provided by you. Right up until the last moments of pregnancy, you are still giving your baby all its nourishment through the umbilical cord – the baby's lifeline from your placenta. For yourself, too, you need good-quality blood to cope with creating this new little person and the inevitable loss of some blood during the birth.

If you are a chesty person or given to sinus or other problems in the respiratory system, you are more vulnerable to anaemia, but you may not realize that this is why you have become more puffed than usual on climbing the stairs or you cannot hold a conversation while walking uphill. Anaemia also puts a strain on your heart as it has to pump harder to get enough oxygen round to the tissues. Heart trouble, such as angina, is worse if you are short of haemoglobin. Both heart and chest disorders – the big killers – are, of course, likelier as we get older. That is why it is so vital to keep your blood in tip-top condition in the Third and Fourth Ages.

While a good supply of oxygen, via the haemoglobin transport system, is important for the smooth functioning of every bodily

4

part, the most delicate of these and the most dependent on oxygen is your brain. It demands a generous supply in order for you to think, feel and remember effectively.

## The Reverend Jeremy

Everyone said it was a tragedy. The Reverend Jeremy J., the erstwhile vicar of St Michael's, was only 71. He had been respected, and well loved, the loving grandfather of young Timothy – until the last 18 months. His personality had changed from benign to bad-tempered and unpredictable, with outbursts of anger and, sometimes, tears. In the evenings especially he seemed barely to know where he was, and the nights were worse: he was restless and noisy, moaning much of the time.

Jeremy was persuaded to resign his living and, sadly, his daughter Judy felt that she could no longer leave him alone with Timothy, whom he had adored. Then the jerky movements – which had gradually started to occur over the months – became incessant. His head, his arms and then all his limbs were involved. His appetite had dwindled to nothing and he had lost weight.

Jeremy's doctor considered two possible diagnoses: Parkinson's disease or arteriosclerotic dementia. Either way, the outlook was grim.

To make sure, the doctor arranged a series of tests. An electroencephalogram (EEG), which is an electrical recording of brain activity, was, as he had feared, abnormal. Then, the result of a routine blood test was surprising. It showed that Jeremy's haemoglobin level was 6.1 – less than half what it should have been, even allowing for his age. His brain was suffering as a result – it could not work properly without enough oxygen, and it was protesting.

A blood transfusion was arranged and 3 pints of blood were used. The results amazed everyone: the jerky movements stopped, Jeremy's tears and rages subsided, and he could think clearly once more. The trace on his EEG reverted to normal. He has not slipped back since.

The cause of Jeremy's anaemia was tracked down to bleeding

piles. Although it had never been noticeably severe, this had had an effect over many years.

Severe anaemia poses a particular risk of being overlooked in cases like Jeremy's because it creeps up so silently. We don't think of anaemia when someone has a serious brain or heart or chest disorder. Perhaps we should. Perhaps the Victorians were right to take anaemia so seriously.

# 2

# Your lifeblood: what it is and what it does

Blood: it is the colour of danger if you spill it, yet the evidence of health in your child's rosy cheeks; it is the very stuff of life. The ancient Hebrews believed that a person's blood contained their soul, which is why the blood is drained out of kosher meat. The Romans thought it carried their most esteemed virtue, courage. Thus, if a valiant warrior was slain, there was competition to drink his blood and so acquire his bravery. Traits of character, good or bad, are still said to be 'in the blood', but nowadays we mean that these are a legacy from our parents, that they are in the genes.

## *What is blood made of?*

Blood consists of a straw-coloured liquid called plasma. It contains three important elements: red blood corpuscles, white corpuscles and myriad minute bodies called platelets.

### *The red cells*

These are the most important, but it wasn't until about 1700 that a Dutchman, Jan Swammerdam, first spotted them with his primitive microscope. 'Ruddy globules' he called them, but no one was interested. In fact, the red cells aren't globular, but an unusual shape: like a disc with the middle part thinner than the edges. This allows them to be squashed into all sorts of shapes without breaking as they are squeezed along the tiniest blood vessels – the capillaries – to take oxygen to the tissues. If they are the wrong size or shape they cannot function properly, and this can cause anaemia.

Ordinarily a healthy red cell lives for 110 days, give or take 3 weeks. This means that there must be a constant replacement system. This applies to the other cells, too.

*Francesca*

Francesca's parents came from Southern Italy, but they had settled in England before she was born because there were better job opportunities for them. She had lived a perfectly healthy life

7

until she was 25, and she got a job as an air hostess. After a few months, she started getting attacks of blood in her urine (quite painless), and she became increasingly tired, easily short of breath and unusually prone to colds and other infections. In spite of eating a good diet, she looked pale. Francesca was found to be anaemic. When her blood was examined under a microscope, a number of her red cells were found to be an odd, new moon shape. These are called sickle cells, and the trait is hereditary. Sickle cell anaemia is commonest in Africa, Arab countries and a few parts of Southern Europe. The sickle-shaped cells tend to get jammed in the blood vessels, and the white cells in the blood then destroy them. The end result is a shortage of red cells and their haemoglobin, that is anaemia. It was the anaemia that made Francesca so tired.

Until she travelled by air regularly, her red cells had been, to all intents and purposes, normal and so she had not been anaemic. However, she carried the hereditary sickle cell trait from her father and this made her red cells vulnerable when she was exposed to the lowering of oxygen levels that occurs at high altitudes. They reacted by turning into the sickle shape. A similar effect could have occurred if she had been given anaesthesia for an operation. Apart from these situations, a carrier of the sickle cell trait usually experiences no problems and may not even be aware of it.

Francesca could not change her heredity, but she could, and did, change her job, and had some short-term treatment for the temporary anaemia in the meanwhile.

## The white cells

These cells come in six forms and are major players in your body's defences. They fend off bacteria, viruses, fungi and parasites that come into the body through your mouth, digestive system, airways, eyes and sexual and urinary openings. The white cells are transported in the blood to wherever there is trouble. They spend up to eight hours circulating in the blood, then four or five days in the affected tissues. Many of them die in the battle with the bugs and the resulting debris is pus. Large numbers of white cells must be produced when there is an infection to deal with, as well as the usual steady replacement of the normal reserves.

### The platelets

These are tiny round or oval discs with a lifespan of two to three weeks. If a blood vessel is damaged – you cut your finger or something worse – some platelets immediately join together to plug the hole. When there is a very small break in the blood vessel this will be enough to stop the blood leaking out; otherwise a clot will form. The platelets play a leading role in this. Healing can go ahead safely when there is no more bleeding.

### Plasma

Plasma is not simply a liquid in which the red and white cells are carried. It contains 7 per cent protein and this is available in the body wherever there is an immediate need (usually about 50g a day are required). In states of shock – for instance after a serious injury or burn – a plasma transfusion can be life-saving, and plasma is easier to keep and transport than whole blood. There is also an effective artificial plasma.

Another function of plasma is that of producing antibodies against specific infections. These are the long-term defences, both during an illness or in prevention, with immunization.

## Where do the solid parts of the blood come from?

As none of the vital blood cells is immortal, a constant manufacturing process has to operate to keep up the supplies. There are urgent calls for extra white cells when there is infection, and for red cells if you become anaemic as a result of a haemorrhage or any other cause. For example, you may move to somewhere like Quito, so high up that the air is thin. During the gold rush to the Andes in the sixteenth century, the European prospectors all became weak and ill, while the local inhabitants were strong and healthy. The newcomers needed time in order for their blood to produce enough red cells to make the best use of the available oxygen.

Unexpectedly, it is a group of cells in the kidneys that monitors the supply of oxygen to the tissues all over the body. These cells produce a hormone – a chemical messenger – that triggers the production of red corpuscles. Damage to the kidneys may interfere with this, which is why people with chronic kidney disease are always anaemic. The control system, as well as ensuring that there are enough red cells, prevents the formation of too many. Otherwise, they could make a dangerous traffic jam in the arteries.

Blood cell production takes place in the liver, spleen and bone marrow in an unborn baby, up until the fifth month of pregnancy. After that, the liver and spleen start to tail off the amount they make and the bone marrow takes over this job entirely. All the bones are involved in this process at birth, but by the age of about 20, it is only the ends of the long bones, ribs, vertebrae and breastbone that still do so. In an emergency, however, the marrow along the whole shaft of the leg and arm bones comes back into service temporarily. Older people have less active bone marrow, so it may barely cover their needs for new blood. Starvation, for instance in anorexia, may also slow down blood production.

## What are the raw materials of blood?

The following are the vital ingredients, and if any of them is in short supply, the body's factories cannot keep up the output required:

- iron;
- protein;
- vitamin C;
- vitamin $B_{12}$;
- folic acid;
- intrinsic factor;
- vitamin $B_6$;
- vitamin E;
- thyroid hormone;
- male hormone (we all have some);
- traces of cobalt and manganese.

### Iron

This is by far the most important raw material and the one most likely to be lacking. Great swathes of the world are subject to iron deficiency – India, Thailand, Cambodia, the Middle East and East

Africa. In the affluent West, vegetarians and those who, like Indian women, eat mainly cooked vegetables and rice, or those old people who live on tea and buns, all have a diet that is inadequate in iron. Diets containing a lot of bread and cereal also contain phytic acid. This prevents your absorbing iron even when it is available. One trap is that wholemeal bread and other whole grain products, which we look upon as being the healthiest, are more damaging in this respect than finely milled white flour. Similarly, white cane sugar, which is anathema to those trying to eat healthily, is excellent at enhancing the uptake of iron. Although it is easy to buy iron tablets to make up any shortfall, your body will not put them to use unless you also have meat in your diet.

In the days of King Arthur and his knights, people believed that if you drank wine in which a hero had steeped his sword, you would become strong: the first iron tonic. By the seventeenth century, they weren't so romantic. A few rusty nails or iron filings in the wine were found to be just as efficacious. No doubt those who, unknowingly, were suffering from iron deficiency anaemia did feel better for the medicine.

Most of the iron in the body is to be found in the haem part of haemoglobin in the red corpuscles – 2.5g out of a total of 4g. If you take in more iron than you require, your body simply discards the surplus in the urine. As the haemoglobin is recycled when worn out red cells are replaced, the body only needs a small amount of iron – say 1mg daily – to keep in balance. There is a small reserve supply in the form of a protein called ferritin, which is in the liver and bone marrow. Some is also circulating in the plasma, but this is reduced during pregnancy, unless you take a supplement.

Iron-containing foods include liver, red meat, dark chocolate, Allbran, sardines, eggs and, among vegetables, spinach, in large quantities.

### Protein

Protein is an essential food, and absolutely necessary for making blood. The globin part of haemoglobin is all protein, and white cells and plasma contain protein, too.

Protein comes from meat, fish, eggs, poultry, cheese, milk, pulses and nuts. Proteins from animal sources, including milk,

11

contain all the vital ingredients for making human protein, but the strictly plant foods do not. This matters a great deal to children as they cannot grow with vegetable protein alone. Some mothers who mistakenly believed that a diet devoid of animal or dairy products, but including plenty of garlic and vegetables, was healthy found their children did not grow normally. You cannot build a child without a supply of top-grade protein, nor can you manufacture blood at any age without it. In fact, making enough haemoglobin is essential to life, and has priority over all the body's other needs when there is a shortage of protein.

### Vitamin C (ascorbic acid)

This is the summertime vitamin – found in salads, raw green vegetables and fresh fruits, with citrus fruits and currants containing the most.

As well as improving the absorption of iron, vitamin C is found in both the blood corpuscles and plasma. A shortage causes the red cells to die early and the small blood vessels to leak (the hallmark of scurvy is bleeding from the gums).

### Vitamin $B_{12}$ (cobalamin)

This vitamin is necessary for the maturing of every cell in the body, but especially those in the blood-forming tissues of the bone marrow. One reason is that it is used in making DNA – the fascinating double spiral that controls every detail of our personal growth and development. In the case of the red blood corpuscles, vitamin $B_{12}$ can only work in conjunction with the intrinsic factor, a substance made in the stomach.

Vitamin $B_{12}$ is unique among the vitamins in that it is not found in any plant. This puts vegans and, to a lesser extent, other vegetarians, at risk of pernicious anaemia and also of disturbances of the nerves and a form of madness, so discussing your diet with a dietitian is therefore essential. Also, children don't grow properly if they do not have an adequate intake of this vitamin. Fortunately, your liver stores a two-year supply of vitamin $B_{12}$ so you need to have a poor diet for a very long time to produce symptoms. In many cases of deficiency, although there is enough of the vitamin in the person's food, they cannot absorb it for some reason.

12

The foodstuffs containing vitamin $B_{12}$ are meat, fish, poultry, eggs and cheese. Milk is the saving grace for the strict vegetarian.

## Folic acid

While ordinarily you have plenty of this vitamin, you need to take supplements of it during pregnancy. Mothers-to-be can become anaemic, especially if they eat a lot of white bread, white rice and other refined and processed foods. Natural sources include liver, spinach, raw broccoli, Brussels sprouts, white fish and wholegrains – and, more exotically, oysters. Folic acid is among the materials needed to make red blood cells.

## Intrinsic factor

This is made by special cells in the lining of the stomach, and is necessary for you to absorb vitamin $B_{12}$, which enables the red blood cells to grow to maturity and do their work. Chronic stomach disease can interfere with the production of intrinsic factor and anaemia will result.

## Vitamin $B_6$ (pyridoxine)

This too, is needed in the making of haemoglobin. The body is seldom short of it because it is in all types of food – meat, vegetables, bread and other cereal foods.

## Thyroid hormone

This promotes the manufacture of all the proteins in the body, including haemoglobin. Too little, as in hypothyroidism, leads to anaemia because production of haemoglobin is then slow and limited. Much too much thyroid hormone also leads to anaemia because it revs up the metabolism and the proteins are then broken down as quickly as they are manufactured.

## Copper, cobalt and manganese

Only a trace of these is needed, and they are to be found everywhere. So, only in very exceptional circumstances can anyone have a deficiency in any of them.

Making blood and its prime component, haemoglobin, is more complicated than cooking a five-star feast – and the process must be continuous – so it is not surprising that now and again things do not run smoothly.

## *Did you know that human haemoglobin can be made by plants?*

In 1997, French research workers found a way of inserting the genes for producing haemoglobin into, of all things, the tobacco plant. The reputation of the, until now, 'evil weed' may be redeemed if it becomes a cheap source of lifesaving haemoglobin, uncontaminated by the AIDS virus or any other harmful organism. The farmers whose livelihood depends on growing tobacco can take heart. As people, wisely, are smoking less and less, there may yet be a really worthwhile market for their crop.

# 3

# The symptoms and signs of anaemia

There is an early warning system that you can easily overlook. The symptoms and signs that should alert you to the possibility that you are suffering from anaemia are deceptively vague. You can easily think of another reason for, say, your feeling washed out, concentration lapsing or having had a few headaches recently. Another snag is that, although there are various types of anaemia, each with a different cause, what you notice is much the same in every case. That is because the basic fault in anaemia is a shortage of haemoglobin, and the effects of this are the same however it has arisen.

*Angela*

Angela was 41. She had just landed a new job as Sister-in-Charge in the Occupational Health Unit. It was a major coup, considering the opposition, and Angela was really keen to do well from the start. The stimulation of the interviews for the post had kept her on top form – until now. Now she felt physically and mentally exhausted. She put this down to being a reaction to the strain she had been under. More worrying – and a major *faux pas* – was getting the name wrong of the woman who was to be her deputy. She would depend on Staff Nurse Jenkinson for local knowledge and, in all probability, the woman already felt sore at not having been appointed to the job herself.

This was not the first time Angela had lost concentration lately or failed to remember some detail. She felt sure that a good night's sleep would put things right, but that seemed to be the one thing she could not achieve. She no longer needed to worry about getting the job, but still she could not relax at night, nor indeed in the day, except in a listless, dispirited sort of way. She couldn't summon up any interest when Lucy, who was 11 now, was bubbling over with what had happened at school. And with John – the most supportive of husbands – Angela could not reciprocate. She could not feel concerned about his difficulties with the Board or find any enthusiasm for sex.

The headaches weren't spectacular, like migraine, but annoyingly throbbing and persistent, mainly at the front. An eye check did not find anything wrong. Although she wasn't anxious about anything, at least not to start with, Angela kept getting little runs of palpitations – thumping heartbeats. They were like what happens in a panic attack, but Angela had nothing to panic about. Now and again she felt rather more out of breath than she expected – when running for a bus or climbing a hill and talking at the same time – but she put that down to being out of condition: she hadn't had the energy to go to the gym or the swimming baths for ages.

Angela wondered if she was becoming neurotic. Nothing seemed to be wrong physically – unless you counted the minor irritation of two of her nails splitting.

You would never have thought of Angela as anaemic – her face was not noticeably pale for a town-dweller – but it was the blood test in the obligatory staff medical that gave it away. She had iron-deficiency anaemia. As a nurse, she ate a sensible diet and she hadn't just had a baby, but the underlying cause had been present for years. She had accepted her rather heavy periods as a matter of course as she had used an intrauterine contraceptive (IUD). Anaemia makes any bleeding worse, so she had been caught in a vicious circle. Treatment with iron tablets brought her haemoglobin up to normal over about eight weeks, and changing to the Pill made her periods shorter and lighter. The IUD was removed.

## Geoffrey

He was a big man: to be honest, he was overweight. He had a demanding job as a quantity surveyor, going round various building sites. He enjoyed his food and plenty of it – sausages and mash, fish and chips, beans on toast or sometimes a Chinese take-away, washed down with strong tea or beer. He often had indigestion, but dealt with it by taking generous doses of an antacid medicine he could buy over the counter. He took it even when his stomach was behaving.

16

It was when he was climbing a ladder at the new power station that a nasty chest pain first caught him. He put it down to his old enemy, indigestion, and doubled the dose of antacid. However, the pain began to crop up quite often, especially when he was doing something energetic.

Geoffrey could see that, at 50, he was a prime candidate for a coronary. His wife, having winkled out what was worrying him, insisted that he see the doctor. An electrocardiogram (ECG) showed that his heart was healthy, but a blood test showed that he was anaemic.

The cause might have been his choice of foods, but dietary analysis ruled that out. What was happening was that the large amounts of antacid Geoffrey had been taking over the last few years were neutralizing the normal acid in his stomach. This meant that he could not produce the vital intrinsic factor necessary for the manufacture of haemoglobin and gradually he had run short, making him anaemic. In fact, Geoffrey had a form of pernicious anaemia.

Geoffrey recovered when he altered his eating habits, stopped taking the indigestion medicine and boosted his vitamin $B_{12}$ stores with injections.

As the effects of anaemia are so unexpected and general, having just one of the symptoms may mean nothing. If, however, you have several of the possible symptoms, you should think that you may have anaemia, and ask your doctor whether or not you should have a blood test. Symptoms to look out for are unusual feelings that you experience, such as pins and needles in your fingers or being short of puff, while there are other signs that you or your doctor, or even a friend, can actually observe.

## Pre-anaemia

Anaemia doesn't suddenly jump out of the blue, short of the emergency situation when you suddenly lose a lot of blood (see page 44). There is a run-up, or prodromal, period. It is essentially a problem that develops slowly and there are three early warning signs:

- poor tolerance of exercise – you can't keep up with the game or the walk like the others and you don't feel well when you exercise;
- your capacity for work – not only the physical kind – nosedives; you don't get things done as you used to do;
- your concentration won't last until you have finished the task in hand or the chapter you are reading and you're less efficient.

Of course, you may have a subclinical viral infection or have missed out on sleep lately, but with either of these the difficulties pass. With pre-anaemia they don't – some of the other symptoms of anaemia take over instead.

## *The symptoms of anaemia*

Here are some of the symptoms you may experience.

- Lack of energy, which you may put down to your age, having a period or a cold.
- Getting tired for no reason, on more than one occasion. It is the effect of not having quite enough oxygen to run your muscles, brain and so on comfortably.
- Shortness of breath when you are going uphill or upstairs or running for a bus, compared with what you used to be able to do. You have to breathe faster to keep the tissues supplied with oxygen as you have less haemoglobin to transport it.
- Palpitations, which is when you feel your heart beating harder and faster. As anaemic blood is less efficient at carrying oxygen, the heart has to pump it round faster.
- Throbbing in your head or ears, which is an effect of the heart's beating harder.
- Chest pain when you take exercise – a form of angina. Your heart muscle is aching like a leg muscle when you have been running hard. In either case the muscle is complaining that it hasn't enough oxygen.
- Dizziness, faintness, which is the effect on your brain when it has too little oxygen.

18

- Headaches, which are also the result of lack of oxygen, similar to the effect of being in a hot, airless room.
- Ringing in the ears – the upset to the nerves and the circulation combine to produce this irritating effect.
- Pins and needles in your hands and feet, which are another effect of lack of oxygen on your nerves.
- Dimness of vision – a faint darkening of the world around, like coming in out of the sun. This, again, is an effect of anaemia on your nerves, in this case the optic nerves conveying vision.
- Poor sleep as it is difficult to settle and you may be restless all night.
- Poor concentration – an effect of anaemia on your brain.
- Low, listless mood: you cannot whip up any interest or enthusiasm. This is sometimes mistaken for postnatal depression if it comes on after having had a baby, but in this case it is due to the loss of blood in childbirth and afterwards.
- A sore, uncomfortable tongue.
- Difficulty in swallowing – a rare effect, only seen in iron-deficiency anaemia.

Sometimes it is the *signs* of anaemia that first make you wonder if something is wrong, or it may be that you or your doctor look for the signs specifically because of symptoms that have aroused your suspicions.

## *The signs of anaemia*

The following are the signs that your doctor will look for.

- Pale skin. Even if it does not show in your face, particularly if you have a dark skin, it may be noticeable in the palms of your hands or in the colour of the nail-bed showing through your fingernails. In some types of anaemia, the pallor has a yellowish tinge.
- Pale mucous membranes, which are the areas of moist skin inside your lips or your eyelids (you can pull the lower one down to look).

- A rapid pulse. Normally it is 80 beats a minute or less. It speeds up as a result of the heart having to pump the blood round faster.
- An enlarged heart.
- Heart murmurs. These and the above are effects of anaemia that your doctor will pick up.
- Swollen ankles, which are an indication that the heart is having to struggle to do more than usual.
- Changes in your nails, such as brittleness, ridging and cracking and a flat appearance. These are signs of iron deficiency, that are sometimes seen in iron deficiency anaemia, but not in other types.
- Cracks and soreness at the corners of the mouth, which are usually found when there is a shortage of iron.

## Emergency symptoms

If you lose a lot of blood suddenly, for instance in a road traffic accident or with a miscarriage:

- your heart beats faster to prevent your blood pressure collapsing;
- your skin is pale, cold and clammy;
- you need to lie flat or you faint.

An ordinarily healthy adult can afford to lose 0.5l (about 1 pint) of blood at any one time without ill effect. This is the amount required from a blood donor. If appreciably more is lost suddenly, you may go into shock. This is an emergency situation, requiring immediate expert assistance from a paramedic or a doctor. A transfusion of blood, plasma or plasma substitute would save your life in this situation. If this were not forthcoming, the body would do its best to produce enough plasma to restore the volume of blood in the course of the next 24–36 hours. The subsequent anaemia, from the loss of red cells in the blood, would take weeks to recover – at best. A transfusion achieves this quickly. However, if there are any problems with iron supplies or there is another illness in the background, chronic anaemia may remain after the acute situation is over.

### Chronic loss of blood

If, for instance, you suffer from piles, heavy periods, other gynaecological problems or a bleeding stomach ulcer, your bone marrow will compensate by increasing the output of new red blood cells. All this extra production drains the body's resources of the raw materials for making blood, particularly iron, and iron deficiency anaemia sets in.

## Investigations when anaemia is suspected

Your doctor may arrange any of the following investigations if there are symptoms and signs of anaemia.

### Preliminary screening

This may include:

- a blood test to include haemoglobin concentration; packed cell volume (PCV; the space in the blood taken up by the red cells); mean red cell haemoglobin (MCH; the average amount of haemoglobin in each red cell);
- a smear test of blood examined under a microscope, showing the size, shape and colour of the red cells and any abnormalities.

### General

In this category would fall:

- X-rays of the chest and digestive system to check for any abnormality that might cause bleeding;
- occult blood test, to check for hidden blood in your motions;
- examination for possible sources of blood loss, such as the reproductive organs and fibroids in women, piles, peptic ulcer, hiatus hernia, inflammation of the gullet.

### Special

This could involve:

- a serum ferritin level check, which is more reliable than a simple iron estimation as ferritin is the storage form of iron in the body: useful when iron deficiency anaemia is suspected;

21

- a serum $B_{12}$ estimation;
- a Schilling test, which is a test for pernicious anaemia (this and a serum $B_{12}$ estimation involve some time and trouble);
- folate level.

## Laura

Laura was nearly 60, just coming up to retirement from her job as School Secretary at the local comprehensive. The school had been her life, and it was not surprising that she should feel down as her time there drew to a close. Since her mother had died, Laura had lived on her own, which didn't help. She hadn't the heart to do much cooking for one and, anyway, because of her sensitive nature, she had become a vegetarian, almost a vegan. It was kinder, natural and less trouble. Besides, if anything, her weight was edging up. She must be eating enough.

As well as feeling down, Laura felt dreadfully weary and cold all the time, and her voice seemed to be permanently hoarse although she hadn't got a cold. However, what caught the doctor's eye was her pale, faintly yellowy complexion.

Blood tests showed that Laura was indeed anaemic, but not with the common iron deficiency type. Nor did tests for the vitamins $B_{12}$ and folate show the shortage the doctor had expected. In view of her sensitivity to cold and her croaky voice, he decided to do a thyroid check. Laura was suffering from hypothyroidism, an underactive thyroid gland. This can be a cause of anaemia in itself. Treatment with thyroxine and a review of her diet improved Laura's health and happiness within weeks.

As in Laura's case, when no obvious deficiency or cause of blood loss can be found to account for anaemia, a general bodily illness may be at the root of the problem. Disorders of the liver, lungs and skin, cancers, rheumatoid arthritis and taking alcohol in excess may all produce anaemia as a complication.

# 4

# Why you may not make enough red cells

Your red blood corpuscles – 'erythrocytes' to give them their medical name – are vital to life and the tissues all over the body depend on them. As red cells wear out in about four months, the bone marrow has to manufacture replacements non-stop. Anything that upsets production means that anaemia and all its consequences are the result.

## *Possible problems with blood cell production*

These include:

- a shortage of the basic ingredients;
- upset to the bone marrow;
- inflammation and infection;
- chronic illness;
- liver and kidney disorders;
- ill effects of certain drugs and medicines;
- faulty genes;
- undue loss of red cells so that replacement cannot keep up.

## *A shortage of the basic ingredients*

The essentials for making blood were given on page 10. The main ingredients for making red blood cells in particular must be provided by your food. They are:

- iron;
- protein;
- vitamin $B_{12}$;
- folate.

## Iron

This is the likeliest ingredient to show a shortfall, although an ordinary healthy diet that includes meat and fresh fruit provides more than enough. Relying on white bread and margarine, buns, crisps, chips and strong tea, however, while filling you up also lets you down nutritionally. Milk doesn't help either, as far as iron is concerned. You might think that a diet of masses of cooked and raw vegetables and fruit, fish but no meat, plus wholemeal bread, oatmeal and brown rice would be good for you. The snag with it, however, is that the phytic acid in the unprocessed cereals kills both the iron and the calcium in your diet. You eat them but you cannot absorb them. The tannin in tea has the same unfortunate effect. Vitamin C, found in oranges and other fresh fruit, and ordinary white sugar and meat protein, on the other hand, help you to absorb as much iron as your body needs.

Top iron-containing foods are liver, red meat, eggs, dried fruit, dark chocolate (not milk or white), Allbran, sardines and real treacle. Green vegetables, like spinach and cabbage, trail behind.

### How much iron do I need?

The people who need most iron are young people of either sex of 12–18 who are growing fast, pregnant women and breastfeeding mothers. All women up to the menopause require more iron than men, while a child between the ages of 7 and 9 uses up as much iron as a man of 35.

### Tests for iron deficiency

Microscopic examination of a blood smear shows pale, undersized red cells, some of them an oval shape, where there is iron deficiency.

Tests on the finger nails show up any long-term shortage of iron.

Chemical tests give the level of iron in the blood.

### How do I overcome iron deficiency anaemia?

Pepping up your iron stores is usually a matter of taking iron tablets (see page 49), but in extreme circumstances an intramuscular injection may be needed.

The tablets can upset an adult's digestive system and bowels, but they can be fatal to a child. Iron pills can look like sweets and are often sugar-coated, so it behoves anyone taking them to keep them safely away from young children.

## Jackie

Jackie was 37 when she had her first child. She had been determined to do everything correctly, the natural way if possible, so was bitterly disappointed when the obstetrician insisted that the birth should be induced ten days early. This had been because of her blood pressure.

Little Anthea – it means a flower – was a beautiful baby: small (2400g, just over 5lbs), but perfect. She was as contented as she was adorable. Even if the birth had not been the easy, natural process Jackie had wanted, feeding Anthea was a complete success. Breast is best – everyone knows that. Jackie had been afraid that she would not be able to supply enough milk, but she and the baby made a winning partnership. Jackie was proud and happy that her baby was having the safest formula, with a built-in boost to her immunity in the early, vulnerable weeks.

Everything seemed to go swimmingly, with mother and baby both enjoying the feeds. Jackie couldn't help feeling gratified when Anthea protested strongly at the first taste of vegetable purée, which she tried at about four months old. She screamed until she was puce. It was clear that this baby did not want any solids when there was delicious, warm, sweet, breast milk on tap. Jackie decided to postpone the introduction of solid foods for a month or two. After all, in some countries, for instance in South America and Africa, mothers go on breastfeeding for as long as two years.

Allowing for the fact of her low birthweight, Anthea had done well in her first two to three months. Looking back, it had started at about the fourth month, very very gradually. Babies' skins are thin and fragile in their first few weeks, but become more substantial – the texture of a rose petal and delicately pink. Anthea's, however, seemed to revert to the early, almost transparent look. She had always been a 'good' baby, not one to scream with rage if bored or hungry or uncomfortable, but

25

Jackie's complacency about this began to be tinged with doubt. It occurred to her, ridiculous though it seemed, that Anthea was too tired to cry. She was not sleeping so well either, but, rather, would lie awake and whimper quietly. She wasn't putting on weight as she should.

Since they had recently moved house, Jackie had not got to know her new medical practice, but she found the doctor there, a woman, helpful and efficient. She took a blood sample quickly and neatly, and was able to tell Jackie that Anthea had iron deficiency anaemia. This is quite common in babies, especially those who arrive early and are small. All babies start with a reserve of iron that they draw on during the first three to four months to make a lot of new red blood cells as they grow, but low birthweight babies use up their store of iron twice as fast and this can leave them depleted. Unfortunately milk, including breast milk, does not provide enough iron on its own. Ordinarily, though, when mixed feeding starts, if meat and vegetable purées are included, the iron store is built up again.

Anthea had started off vulnerable, because of her small size, and the delay in starting mixed feeding had made matters worse. However, a change of regime and extra iron brought the pink hue of health back to her skin and she had the energy to make more fuss!

### Protein

This is necessary for all bodily building and repair work, including red cell replacement. It is also the fuel for energy.

The very best foods for providing protein are lean beef, dried and fatty fish, soya, beans and peas, eggs, nuts and skimmed milk. A varied mixture of different kinds of protein food is the most beneficial, and children and pregnant mothers require that a part of their protein intake comes from an animal source (see pages 11–12).

### Vitamin B₁₂ (cobalamin)

This unusual vitamin is involved in the making of DNA, the chemical spiral which carries the complicated genetic code that controls the growth and development of every part of the body, including the bone marrow where the red cells are made and even the red cells themselves. During the course of a pregnancy the growing baby draws on the mother's plentiful store of vitamin $B_{12}$. Thus her supplies are gradually reduced while the baby's are built up. By the time the baby is born, it has more vitamin $B_{12}$, proportionately, than the mother.

Cobalamin is found in all the animal foods you eat, from milk to eggs to meat, but there is none in fruits and vegetables (vegetarians and vegans should therefore consult with a dietitian). It can only be absorbed when it is attached to the intrinsic factor in the stomach (see page 13). Any condition that impedes the production of intrinsic factor, therefore, means that there will be a shortfall in the amount of vitamin $B_{12}$ that you absorb. Problems that have this effect include gastritis, stomach operations and autoimmune disorders. The latter are when errors are made in identification by the defence system, so that the body turns against some of its own cells as though they were invading bacteria, and makes antibodies against them. Autoimmune diseases that may interfere with the body's manufacturing cobalamin are pernicious anaemia (when the cells making intrinsic factor are specifically targeted), thyroid disorders and diabetes. Liver and pancreas problems and diverticulosis (a common age-related condition of the colon) can also prevent the body's making use of the cobalamin available, and so lead to a deficiency anaemia.

*Tests for vitamin $B_{12}$ deficiency*

Microscopic examination of the blood shows extra large red cells, of all different sizes and shapes, when there is a shortage of vitamin $B_{12}$.

The amount of vitamin $B_{12}$ in the blood can also be measured (see page 60).

**Folate (folic acid)**

Unlike cobalamin, this vitamin is present in generous amounts in green vegetables as well as liver, kidney and yeast extracts, such as Marmite.

At birth, the amount of folic acid in the red cells is at an all-time high, but it falls to a low by three months because a milk diet provides hardly any. For this reason, and because milk is also lacking in iron, it is important to introduce meat and vegetable purées soon after starting mixed feeding at four months. Too long on a milk diet, including breast milk, can check a child's growth. Goat's milk is the worst milk to give young children because it is also low in vitamin $B_{12}$.

While a large reserve of cobalamin is stored in the liver, this is not the case with folate. Mothers-to-be, especially when planning to conceive, in the first three months and in the last six months of pregnancy, and mothers who are breastfeeding need a diet rich in folate, or folic acid, and taking a supplement in tablet form is advised. Those with liver disorders, rheumatoid arthritis, on kidney dialysis or who drink heavily also require extra folic acid.

Like vitamin $B_{12}$, folate is needed for making DNA and a shortage interferes with the production of red blood cells. When there is deficiency, under a microscope the blood is similar to that of a person with cobalamin deficiency. Sometimes vitamin $B_{12}$ and folate are *both* in short supply – for instance in a heavy drinker who doesn't bother to eat properly.

## Bob

It was Evelyn who was worried. Bob, like a good many husbands, was not interested in health, and certainly not his own. The insurance medical was the first time he had seen a doctor since he'd broken his ankle skiing. It came as a surprise to him when the doctor told him he had high blood pressure and should do something about it. His own GP said that, at 54, it made sense to have a thorough check-up, but an examination showed nothing apart from the high blood pressure, and that could be controlled. All he had to do was to take one little tablet every morning: one of the water tablets (diuretics) that did not require him to take extra potassium. It seemed to suit Bob: he had none of the possible side-effects, such as nausea, diarrhoea or headaches, and it kept his blood pressure in check.

About 18 months later, Evelyn said she didn't think Bob looked very healthy. Bob had always had rather a red face, but now it was more of a putty colour and he seemed to have lost some of his accustomed energy and enthusiasm for things. He was drinking a little more than usual, but then he had always enjoyed his whisky and he never got drunk. Evelyn kept telling him that he ought to have another check-up, but he brushed her anxieties aside until two things happened: his golf handicap went up and he fell asleep at a Board meeting.

Bob was found to be anaemic. The blood tests showed that he wasn't short of iron or vitamin $B_{12}$, but he was low in folate. When looked at under the microscope, some outsize red cells were found. His doctor put him on a course of folate tablets (it would have been dangerous to do this if he had not already checked that Bob's blood contained plenty of vitamin $B_{12}$). He also suggested that if Bob must drink, he should change from whisky to wine or beer.

The explanation for Bob's anaemia was a fairly unusual effect of the diuretic pills in conjunction with regular doses of alcohol, combining to deplete his blood of folate. His preference for spirits and for cooked food rather than salads and fruit did not help him.

## Inflammation and infection

Viral illnesses, such as shingles, measles, glandular fever and influenza, can sometimes cause haemolysis, which is the leakage of haemoglobin out of the red blood cells into the surrounding plasma, where it cannot transport oxygen to the tissues. In malaria, a particular kind of autoimmune haemolysis can be very serious. Iron is not absorbed properly during an acute illness and there is sometimes a loss of blood as a result of slight bleeding in the digestive system that goes unnoticed, or a more obvious nosebleed. All of these effects make anaemia likely, which is why it is important to allow yourself time for convalescence with good, nourishing food.

Inflammatory disorders of the digestive system itself, such as gastritis, inflammation of the gullet or a hiatus hernia, or inflammation of the colon can lead to a steady seeping away of blood or frank bleeds, darkening the motions, and producing anaemia. If the stomach itself or the bowels are involved, there may also be a shortage of vitamin $B_{12}$ or folate.

29

## Chronic illness

Mild to moderately severe anaemia is a common occurrence after about two months of many illnesses. Examples are rheumatoid arthritis, widespread eczema or psoriasis, tuberculosis, lupus, lung cancer or polymyalgia rheumatica. In fighting the illness, extra folate is used, often leaving a deficiency, which means that red cell production is impaired. If iron is poorly absorbed, there may be a lack of that also.

Anaemia may develop so insidiously that it becomes severe enough to put a strain on the heart and the first indication of trouble is incipient heart failure. The symptoms are a feeling of exhaustion, shortness of breath and a tendency for the ankles to swell.

## Liver and kidney disorders

In viral hepatitis, the red blood cells die early and there is occasionally haemolysis (leakage of haemoglobin fom the red cells). Anaemia results if there are not enough of the materials available nor sufficient time to replace the cells as quickly as they disappear. In cirrhosis of the liver, there is deficiency of both iron and folate as well as haemolysis, producing a form of anaemia in which the red cells are overly large – macrocytic anaemia.

The kidneys manufacture epo (erythropoietin), a hormone that triggers the bone marrow to make haemoglobin for the red cells. When the kidneys are not working properly, they do not make enough epo and, in addition, poisons accumulate in the bloodstream, interfering with the blood-manufacturing process. Iron and folate stores fall away, also inhibiting normal red cell production.

## Ill effects of certain drugs and medicines

### Excessive intake of alcohol

Alcohol is a socially accepted drug and, taken in excess, a general poison, upsetting the metabolism in several ways. Around 50 per cent of heavy drinkers are anaemic, partly because of the direct effect of the alcohol on the blood-forming tissues, and on the survival of the red cells. There is usually a lack of folate, especially in drinkers of spirits (wine is little better, but beer is actually rich in folate). Because bleeding from the digestive tract is common among alcoholics, many also become iron-deficient and have a mixed anaemia, lacking in both iron and folate.

## The effects of medicines

A large number of prescription drugs may occasionally cause haemolysis and anaemia, often when the drug has been used quite safely previously. Examples are ibuprofen, used in the treatment of rheumatic pain; chlorpropamide and glibenclamide, taken for diabetes; erythromycin and benzyl penicillin, antibiotics; cimetidine, taken for peptic ulcers; various antihistamines; sulpha drugs; carbamazepine, an anticonvulsant; tetracycline, and others. The effects are due to the people taking the drugs being particularly sensitive. Some antimalarial medicines can cause a particular kind of haemolysis – and anaemia, which has the same symptoms, however it is produced.

Another group of medicines can sometimes interfere with the metabolism of folate or vitamin $B_{12}$ and lead to anaemia of the macrocytic (big red cell) type. Examples include phenytoin and primidone, both anti-epileptics; and, less commonly, sulphasalazine, used in the treatment of ulcerative colitis; triamterene, a water tablet; or the oral contraceptives.

Some drugs, such as indomethacin, fenoprofen and gold salts, used mainly in the treatment of rheumatoid arthritis, and carbamazepine and chlorpropamide, mentioned above, occasionally have a direct inhibitory effect on the making of red blood cells. Fortunately, these side-effects of medicines are unusual, but should be borne in mind when there is no other explanation for anaemia.

# Faulty genes

Some forms of anaemia are hereditary. Some of them cause a lack of certain enzymes that are necessary to make normal, healthy, red blood cells and normal haemoglobin.

Sickle cell anaemia is common throughout Africa, but is also found in the Middle East and Mediterranean countries and some parts of India, and, of course in people emigrating from these areas. The anaemia is caused by a leakage of haemoglobin from the sickle-shaped red blood corpuscles.

Thalassaemia – either the alpha type, which is mild, or the beta type, which is severe – is similar to sickle cell anaemia and is seen mainly in the same areas, but it occurs in all racial groups. In both types of the condition, the carriers of the faulty gene are resistant to malaria and are not themselves anaemic, but it is particularly important to identify carrier mothers in pregnancy, so that they may be counselled.

Another important enzyme, G6PD, may be genetically deficient. G6PD deficiency makes the sufferers vulnerable to haemolysis if they use any of a wide range of medicines that are ordinarily safe or eat broad beans. Only males are affected, but mothers may be carriers of the gene.

The hereditary anaemias are not common in Northern Europe or North America, but may appear in those whose parents came from Africa, Asia or the Mediterranean borders.

## Undue loss of red cells

Apart from the hereditary disorders and the effects of some medicines, autoimmune antibodies can mistakenly attach themselves to the red cells and cause haemolysis in the course of several illnesses. These include influenza, measles, chicken pox, shingles, listeria infection, glandular fever, viral pneumonia and cirrhosis of the liver. Various poisons, such as snake venom, have a directly damaging effect on the cells, as do particular organisms, such as staphylococci, which lurk on the skin and can cause abscesses, haemolytic streptococci which cause tonsillitis, and the malaria parasite. Severe burns have the same effect (see page 86).

The commonest reason of all for losing red cells is bleeding, either obvious or hidden, in which case it is most likely to come from the digestive system or, in women, through the vagina (see page 47).

*Ashley, Shaun and Sam*

These three friends shared a tatty flat in Kennington. They were students at university in London and not wealthy. There were so many new and exciting things to do in the metropolis now that they were away from their parents, at any rate in term time, that funds were always short. Food was not something they spent much money on. Porridge, bread, cheese, cornflakes and milk were all useful fillers, and all lacking in iron.

The group partied often, especially at weekends when they sometimes took Speed or Ecstasy to keep themselves awake. Oddly enough, lack of sleep leads to there being lower levels of iron in the blood – until the sleep deficit is restored. Sam, unlike Ashley and Shaun, had the added monthly drain on her blood supply and, specifically, the valuable red cells and their iron when she had her period, but they were all, at 18 to 20, still needing maximum amounts of iron as the boys were still growing and this would probably continue until they were nudging 21. They were all on the borderline of needing extra iron supplies at just the wrong time in their lives. With better luck they would probably have got by with no more than a few waves of the deadly fatigue and long, deep sleeps that characterize adolescence.

One day in March, Shaun became ill. He felt, as he said, flaked out, he didn't want to eat, his head ached and his throat hurt. That evening he was boiling hot. One of their friends, who was a medical student, diagnosed tonsillitis and said Shaun ought to have an antibiotic. Sam, fortunately it seemed, had a few amoxycillin capsules left over from a chest infection she'd had at Christmas. Shaun started taking these and promptly developed a rash: he was obviously no better. When Shaun went to see his doctor he thought Shaun had infectious mononucleosis – glandular fever – as he had seen several other students with it. He stopped the antibiotic. Just over a week later, Sam went down with the illness – hers started with a nasty nosebleed. Ashley escaped it altogether.

Shaun recovered quite quickly but Sam continued to feel weak and dizzy and she looked like a ghost. This went on for

33

several weeks with no improvement, until finally the doctor arranged for her to have a blood test. Sam was found to have iron deficiency anaemia. There were several reasons for this. First, there was her age, one when there was an especial need for iron. Then there was the poor diet she and the boys were having, low in iron, vitamin C and protein – all necessary for making red blood cells. The Speed and E, although she had not taken much, may have had a toxic effect on her bone marrow, but this was not very likely. The real precipitating factor was the glandular fever, an infection often associated with anaemia and one adolescents and young adults are particularly prone to. Nosebleeds and the appearance of blood in the urine, if they occur, are only part of the cause: the illness itself leads to anaemia.

One of the tricky things about anaemia is that it can develop when you are distracted by the presence of another illness, as with Sam and her glandular fever.

# 5

## Iron deficiency anaemia

Iron is an essential constituent of the body, amounting to 4–5g altogether. Most of this is in the haemoglobin of the red blood cells, and nearly all the rest is in store in the liver and bone marrow where it is called on for making new blood. Anaemia that arises due to a shortage of iron is a common, worldwide form of ill health. The likeliest cause of it is loss of blood, including the iron it contains. Women in particular are affected because of their vulnerable reproductive system. From their first period, at $12\frac{3}{4}$, give or take a year or two, there is a monthly loss, then, during pregnancy, there is the huge demand by the baby during the last four or five months, topped off by a considerable loss of blood during the birth and afterwards. Men, in days gone by, often lost blood as a result of war wounds when the weapons were swords and spears, but now they do not suffer the same kinds of losses that women do simply living their normal lives.

Anaemia must always have been around, but it was not recognized and given a name until 150 years ago. Earlier than that, however, in Europe, from the seventeenth century, a condition called 'chlorosis' was causing concern. It affected adolescent girls and young women and their complexions were so pale and washed out that they looked faintly greenish. They were noted to suffer from palpitations and become breathless and exhausted at the slightest effort – even just climbing the stairs. They had no appetite. Because of their age and sex, it was all put down to love-sickness, but the general strengthening medicine given – iron filings in wine – seemed to help. With hindsight we can see that they had iron deficiency anaemia. Less helpful than the fortified wine, however, was the fact that the favourite remedy at that time, for almost any ailment, from smallpox to hysteria, was blood-letting. No doubt this was excellent for the overweight, overfed men with high blood pressure, but it would definitely have been damaging to an anaemic young girl. Another popular treatment was cupping, an alternative method of inducing bleeding, or clusters of blood-sucking leeches were applied. Purging accompanied everything else, adding to the weakening effect by reducing the amount of protein, but there was a theory around that most illnesses, including chlorosis, were caused by old food going bad in the colon.

These 'cures' remained in use until nearly the end of the last century. The only sensible idea the doctors had was that diet might be involved in chlorosis. Men ate a lot more than women – especially meat – and they did not suffer from chlorosis. The Victorian miss was told that meat was 'too stimulating' for a nicely brought up young lady. No wonder so many women died in childbirth, drained of their reserves. Another theory was that tight lacing caused chlorosis, and certainly young women were always interested in fashion. Loosening the stays may not have helped the anaemia, but it must have been a relief none the less.

The breakthrough came in 1895. Dr Stockman recognized that the type of anaemia so common both in England and on the Continent was due to a shortage of iron. Treatment with iron pills was, and is, rational and effective. Nevertheless, iron deficiency anaemia has not been banished. It is endemic among women in large swathes of Asia, the Middle East and East Africa, especially among those who live on unprocessed grain. Even in the affluent West, it is still common and often goes unrecognized. In the United Kingdom the black spots are in South Wales and North-West Scotland, where the iron intake may be only half the healthy minimum.

## Spot the enemy: how can you detect iron deficiency anaemia?

The general symptoms of anaemia are listed in full on pages 18–19 and 19–20. If you are experiencing more than one of these, this should alert you at once, but there are also some that only crop up in iron deficiency anaemia, affecting various parts of the body.

### Outward appearances

Everyone expects people with anaemia to look pale, but skin colour can be deceptive. It doesn't only depend on the amount of haemoglobin in your blood – your circulation has a big effect. Even an anaemic person can blush or go pink with heat or exercise. However, there are two places where you can sometimes see the paleness of the blood itself. First, there are the creases in the palms of your hands – your heart line, life line and the others. These are normally pinker than the surrounding skin if you stretch them open. Second, look at the colour of the flesh that shows through underneath your finger nails: it will be paler than the surrounding skin. This is a particularly useful check if you have dark skin.

### *Mucous membranes*

These comprise the moist, delicate lining of your mouth, lips and eyelids, and other parts, like the inside of your stomach, which are out of sight. It is traditional for the doctor to pull down your lower eyelid to see if it looks pale, but this test only works if the haemoglobin level in the blood is 9g/dl or less. The lowest figure regarded as normal is 11.5 for a woman, 13.5 for a man, so mild to moderate anaemia won't show up in the colour of your eyelid.

When the anaemia is due to a lack of iron, the membranes lining the mouth, stomach and intestines become thinner and more fragile. This may disturb your digestion, but, more importantly, it can prevent the absorption, not only of iron itself, but also of vitamin $B_{12}$. A lack of this vitamin causes another type of anaemia, and you can have both kinds at once. Part of the effect of iron deficient anaemia on the membranes is the uncomfortable and unsightly symptom: angular stomatitis. This is redness, soreness and cracking at the corners of the mouth. It occurs more often in women, particularly when the person has dentures that don't fit very snugly.

The tongue is often affected, especially in older people. The tiny papillae which give the tongue its rough appearance all but disappear, leaving the surface looking oddly bald. There may be one or two deep fissures, but they don't hurt and you can still taste your food properly.

### *The finger nails*

These are particularly sensitive to a shortage of iron. The first thing you may notice is that they have become rather brittle, splitting and cracking at the edges. Sometimes there are ridges running towards the tips, and these tend to split. The next stage is when the whole nail becomes flat instead of curving to the shape of your finger, and it looks curiously dry and dead. Finally, koilonychia may develop. This term means 'spoon-shaped', and the nail actually becomes concave instead of convex. The nails provide a measure of how much iron there is in the body as a whole, and nail clippings can be analysed in a laboratory to see what the level is. A total of less than 4muG per gram of nail constitutes deficiency.

## The Hair

Like the nails, your hair can provide a measure of your health. In iron deficiency anaemia, hair becomes thinner and breaks more easily.

## Difficulty swallowing

This manifests as a feeling of there being 'something in the way' when you swallow. It is uncommon and affects mainly middle-aged women. It is due to a thin web of tissue partially blocking the gullet just past the voice-box, and is part of the general upset to the lining membranes brought about by anaemia.

This symptom has two names because doctors found it so interesting that they wanted their own names attached to it. It is called the Plummer-Vinson or the Patterson-Kelly syndrome. It never completely prevents swallowing and things return to normal when the anaemia is treated.

## Disturbed vision

In very severe iron deficiency anaemia – particularly if it has come on rapidly, for instance with the loss of blood due to exceptionally heavy periods – there may be several small haemorrhages in the retina at the back of the eye. This is a rare occurrence and is treated with lasers.

## Geraldine

Geraldine was 69. On retiring from her job as Senior Tutor (Biology) at a women's college, she had taken a keen interest in the local literary group, the Friends of St Martha's Hospital and the Natural History Society. Like many older women academics, she made no concessions to fashion. The effect was a general lack of colour, with an accent, if any, on beige: skirt, blouse and cardigan. She wore no make-up on her pale face, and her wispy hair was cut like a schoolgirl's.

She would have told you that she was perfectly well thank you (except for her teeth), but of course you couldn't expect to stay young forever. She was slowing down and seemed to get tired at the slightest exertion. She had endured a lot of dental trouble lately. The lower set in particular was slopping about in her mouth, making it awkward to eat properly. If she was with other people she certainly could not risk trying anything with pips or that needed chewing, so she tended to stick to soup, mash, porridge and cake. At home she dunked her biscuits. None of this provided her with iron. To make matters worse, she had developed these sore places at the corners of her mouth – little raw cracks that made it uncomfortable to open her mouth at all wide. She did not feel it was right to bother the doctor with something so trivial. Nor did she think it justifiable to mention the tingling she had been getting in her fingers lately. It was like the feeling you get when you warm your hands by the fire when they've gone dead with cold.

It was the difficulty with swallowing, though, that frightened her. Geraldine was sure, immediately, that it was cancer. She imagined the tumour swelling in her throat and choking her. She could feel something in her gullet, just below her voice-box. Because of her independent outlook, Geraldine scarcely knew her doctor, but she seemed concerned and interested and examined her thoroughly. She could see nothing abnormal at the back of Geraldine's throat, but she noticed her poor colour. Both her skin and lower eyelids were unusually pale. Her pulse rate – 95 per minute – was unduly fast considering that she had been sitting chatting to her for the past ten minutes. The doctor also thought she could detect a hint of swelling round Geraldine's ankles.

She arranged a routine blood test and a barium swallow. For the latter, Geraldine went to the hospital. There she had to drink a glass of thick, white, pepperminty liquid while they did an

X-ray. The reports of the results of each test came back just over a week later, and Geraldine, with her scientific training, was keen to see them and have them explained. Her doctor was delighted to have such an interesting case and agreed willingly. She told Geraldine that she had severe iron deficiency anaemia, and that her sore mouth, lack of zest and the swallowing problem were all part of it. The results of the blood test were the evidence of this:

- Hb (haemoglobin) 8.1g/dl – normal for a woman is 13.5–15.5g/dl;
- RBC (red blood corpuscles) 4.1 millions per ml – normal is 3.9–5.6 millions per ml;
- PCV (packed cell volume) 26.8 per cent – normal is 36–48 per cent;
- MCV (mean corpuscular volume) 65fl – normal is 86–95fl;
- MCH (mean corpuscular haemoglobin) 19.6pg – normal is 27–34pg.

These results showed that Geraldine's blood was deficient in haemoglobin, although she had a normal number of red cells. The proportion of her blood comprising cells in relation to the fluid plasma (PCV) was well below normal, because her red cells were undersized (MCV). They also contained less haemo-globin in each (MCH), even allowing for their size. This picture of small red cells containing too little haemoglobin is typical of iron deficiency anaemia. As the iron in the blood is nearly all in the haemoglobin, there was no need in this case to do a separate estimation of the iron content of her blood. A blood smear confirmed the situation, showing the small pale cells, some of them oval and other odd shapes.

The barium swallow X-ray showed that there was a fragile web of lining tissue interfering with the free passage of food down the gullet (oesophagus), typical of the Plummer-Vinson syndrome. This is an uncommon complication of iron deficiency anaemia and so Geraldine's doctor referred her to a consultant haematologist, which is a doctor who is a specialist in blood disorders. The treatment began with an iron injection, rather than the standard tablets.

# What does it feel like to be anaemic?

The general symptoms of anaemia – all types – are listed in full on pages 18–19, and all are due to a shortage of haemoglobin, however this has been caused. The result of this is that the blood the heart must pump round to supply the tissues is substandard.

The basic overriding symptom of iron deficiency, as in other forms of anaemia, is the effort required to get through a normal day, a feeling of lassitude before you begin and fatigue before you are halfway through. Your brain demands a steady, adequate supply of oxygen and if it is short-changed you feel fuzzy, dizzy and headachey. You may even faint, and poor vision can be a part of the problem, too. Your concentration is non-existent.

The knock-on effect of poor-quality blood on your heart and circulation forces the heart to speed up, and this can give you palpitations in your chest and throbbing in your head and ears. Secondarily, as your heart gets tired from all the racing, you are likely to get short of breath with any extra exertion and, perhaps, experience pains in your chest, swollen ankles or ringing in your ears.

Unless you are especially geared to think of anaemia, it isn't the first explanation for these problems that comes to mind. You may fear that you have got a genuine heart or chest disease. The headaches, if they persist, can put the thought of a brain tumour into your mind, and the woolly thinking and loss of concentration you experience may convince you that you have early Alzheimer's disease. Claire, for example, doing her A levels, found she was reading the same paragraph over and over and was still not absorbing it. Black coffee did not help. Claire decided that she was just naturally dim, yet she was at the peak age for anaemia.

# Anaemia and children

### Babies

An anaemic mother starts her baby at a disadvantage, so the custom of taking an iron supplement during pregnancy is really important. Babies need a high level of haemoglobin – and iron – when they enter the world, as they readily become anaemic, whether fed

41

breast milk or formula. They are especially vulnerable, as we have seen, if they are naturally small when they are born or born premature and, in any case, if introducing a mixed diet is delayed much after the age of four months. The very best of milk does not provide a growing baby with adequate quantities of iron. Weaning foods should include puréed meat and green vegetables, plus orange juice, which helps in the absorption of iron.

Indications that a baby is short of iron are undue lack of activity, poor appetite, a quiet whininess and failure to put on adequate weight. Your health visitor or doctor will work out what the problem is and suggest the best treatment.

## *Older children*

They, too, may become anaemic. Their reaction is seldom what you would expect. Rather than sitting quietly, looking sorry for themselves, they are likely to get into trouble at school for being inattentive, show no motivation for work, but wear everyone out by being hyperactive. They also tend to catch any illness that is around. There is no intellectual liveliness, such as most children have, yet an anaemic child may have a perfectly good brain. It is simply being starved of the generous supplies of oxygen and haemoglobin that are needed in increasing quantities up to the age of 20. Iron is necessary to make the haemoglobin that carries the oxygen to the brain as elsewhere.

Badly behaved children always need to be regarded with suspicion – suspicion, that is, that there is an illness underlying the mischief. One curious habit, which may arise when a child has iron deficiency anaemia, and be mistaken for naughtiness is called pica. It comprises eating inappropriate materials like coal, sand or a diet of nothing but peanuts.

## *Jonathan*

Aged six, Jonathan was the bane of his mother's, and his teacher's, life. He was always into something undesirable or dangerous, seemed incapable of sitting still for five minutes and was making no progress at school. He wasn't interested on the one hand, and on the other, he didn't remember what he had

42

been told from one minute to the next. It was partly due, his teachers thought, to his missing so much school. It seemed as though he was never without a runny nose or a cough. His resistance to infection was so poor, and his appetite was non-existent.

His Gran told Jonathan that he would never be big and strong like Popeye if he didn't eat up his healthy meat and greens, but he just didn't feel hungry. An odd thing – which made his mother take him to the doctor yet again – was that she had found him eating earth, cramming it into his mouth as though it were food. The doctor said this was pica and explained. It can happen in children with severe learning difficulties or pregnant women, but Jonathan was neither of these. It doesn't always involve something as weird as earth or coal or wood, but may appear like an exaggerated craze for a particular food, such as peanuts or eggs. Children who are short of calcium have been known to eat the plaster off the wall, but those deprived of sufficient iron may eat almost anything unusual. Adults with iron deficiency can develop pica, too. Jonathan had iron deficiency anaemia and, with treatment, his transformation into a normal little boy was a slow miracle.

*Alice*

She was a perfectly sensible woman of 50, but had an overwhelming desire for carrots. Indeed, she ate so many that she developed a slightly orange hue to her skin and her general nutrition suffered. She, like Jonathan, had iron deficiency anaemia. Iron replacement cured Alice of this peculiar symptom.

## Doctors' tests

With any of the signs or symptoms described, it is essential to consult your doctor. He or she can set in motion some of the following definitive tests, as appropriate:

- blood count, to check your haemoglobin level and the state of your red blood cells;

- blood smear test, to assess the look of your red cells in particular – a haematologist can recognize blood disorders as easily as you can recognize a friend's face;
- radio-iron test, to check if iron is being absorbed properly;
- serum iron estimation, to check if there is the normal amount of iron in your blood;
- urinary iron, to see if you are losing too much by this route;
- occult (meaning 'hidden', nothing sinister) blood test, to see if you are losing blood from the digestive tract;
- X-ray of your chest and neck, to check just in case there are lung or thyroid problems.

## *The three commonest causes of iron deficiency anaemia*

These are:

- loss of blood, which automatically means loss of iron;
- an inadequate diet (see page 48);
- malabsorption.

Any of these is more serious if it arises in one of the periods of life when you are naturally particularly vulnerable to this type of anaemia. These times are:

- from six months onwards as a baby;
- as a fast-growing adolescent;
- during pregnancy and the birth and a little afterwards;
- to a mild extent, if you are a woman, until the menopause;
- in later life, as the bone marrow hasn't the resilience to make up for any losses quickly.

### *Loss of blood*

Far the commonest cause of iron deficiency anaemia is loss of blood, with its valuable content of iron-containing haemoglobin. Although your body carefully recycles the haemoglobin from the worn out blood cells that have come to the end of their life, it can do nothing about blood that is actually spilt or red cells that break inside the blood vessels. The iron is more difficult to replace than the protein part of the haemoglobin, which the body can make up from its internal resources, but the iron reserve in the bone marrow is quickly used up when there is an extra call on it to make new blood.

Some blood losses are normal. Women lose blood every month. In an ordinary monthly period, you lose a total of 20–40mg of iron. This means that you need to take in and absorb at least 2mg of iron daily instead of the basic 1–1.5mg required by men, children and those past the menopause. Paradoxically, if you are anaemic already, you tend to lose even more blood than usual with each period.

Having a baby is normal, too, and a dramatic drain on a mother-to-be's iron supplies, the amount it takes from her escalating from the twenty-fourth week of pregnancy on. All-in-all a baby demands between 400 and 500mg of iron during the time it depends on its mother's blood for everything it needs. Over the course of the nine months of pregnancy, this averages out at double the mother's usual requirement, despite her having no periods. It is therefore easy to see that there is usually an urgent need to take iron tablets during this time (see page 24).

The birth itself and the time a little while afterwards deplete the mother's reserves of another 300mg, and possibly much more if it is a difficult birth.

Breastfeeding also calls for an extra 0.5mg of iron a day, over and above the basic requirement, depending on when periods start up again.

Blood donation, although not exactly normal, isn't an illness either. If you donate 2 pints of blood during the year, you must absorb an extra 1mg of iron daily throughout those 12 months. You cannot replace the iron as quickly as you can give it away.

Joggers and competition runners are healthy, but 50 per cent of them experience temporary anaemia. Probably all that is needed is to make sure that they eat a good mixed diet.

*Amy*

Amy and Tim were among the happiest couples you could imagine, until the twins came. Amy had been an only child and always said that she wanted a 'real family' with four children, two boys and two girls.

They lived on the outskirts of a country town, ideal for children, while Tim found it well worth commuting to his job in the City. Money wasn't flowing, but it was enough. There was no financial reason for not putting their plan for a family into operation. At 24 and 28 respectively, Amy and Tim had achieved their dream of having four children – Tim junior was 4, Edward $2\frac{1}{2}$, and the twins, identical girls, were 15 months old.

Amy had a mother's help, a treasure who took a lot of the physical chores off her shoulders, and Tim pulled his weight at weekends. Even so, Amy couldn't enjoy her little ones or, indeed, anything about her life. She was unreasonable with the helper and edgy with Tim, sex was a thing of the past and nothing seemed worth the bother. Amy had lost her appetite and her hair was a mess, with no spring or shine. The world, as she saw it, seemed to be literally tinged with grey.

Amy was anaemic. She had taken her iron and folic acid tablets religiously during the pregnancies, but that hadn't been enough. The four babies had come too close together, and the final straw was having the twins. Each over 2.8kg (6lbs) at birth, they had made enormous inroads into Amy's iron stores and, to cap it all, she decided to have a try at breastfeeding them. Six weeks of this exhausted her completely and she was forced to give up. Amy's doctor gave her one iron injection, tablets for a whole year and strict instructions to have no more babies without having a blood test first!

Sudden, severe blood loss may occur if you are unlucky enough to be involved in a terrible motorway pile-up or an industrial accident. A varicose vein may bleed alarmingly after a trivial knock; you may have a miscarriage; or you may have embarrassing flooding around the time of the menopause. All these are emergency situations, requiring urgent medical or paramedical attention (see page 60). There will also be a need for follow-up treatment with iron pills for many months to restore the lost blood and the health that goes with it.

Chronic blood loss is by far the commonest and most often neglected reason for the development of iron deficiency anaemia.

46

This is because the bleeding is likely to be so slight as to be ignored or to go unrecognized, although it takes the loss of only a teaspoonful of blood daily for anaemia to occur eventually. This is because the balance between loss and restoration dips just to the wrong side.

The area of the body most prone to silent, unseen bleeding is the digestive tract, from mouth to anus. You can have bleeding gums at one end or piles, internal or external, at the other. The oesophagus (swallowing tube) can become inflamed and ooze blood as food passes down, particularly if there is a hiatus hernia to impede the steady progress into the stomach, which has a tougher lining than the oesophagus. The pleasantly warm sensation when brandy or other strong drink goes down is an indication of its actually irritating the lining membrane *en route*. This is why heavy drinkers tend to develop varicose veins in the oesophagus, and these are much more delicate than if they occur elsewhere. A serious haemorrhage of one can result from trivial damage.

Similarly, if the stomach or duodenum become ulcerated, perhaps due to the helicobacter bug that settles in this area, a slight but continuous loss of blood may result. Even more likely (and probably the commonest cause of iron deficiency anaemia in the UK) is bleeding in the stomach because of the irritation to the lining brought about by painkillers such as aspirin or the anti-inflammatories (NSAIDs), used to treat arthritis and rheumatic pain. There may be stomach pain as well as bleeding, and this can be alleviated to some extent by adding another medicine. Steroid medication – used in the treatment of asthma and other illnesses – can have a similar effect on the stomach. The bleeding will not be enough to make a noticeable difference to the colour of the motions, but enough to cause anaemia.

An occult blood test (see page 44) will detect traces of altered blood in the stools and is a standard investigation when anaemia is suspected. It will, of course, also pick up evidence of any bleeding lower down the digestive tract, for instance if there are polyps in the colon, cancer or the common, age-related condition of diverticulosis. Diverticulosis is when little pouches have developed in the walls of the colon, and these tend to get inflamed and bleed a little.

Women's reproductive systems readily bleed for a variety of reasons – from psychological stress to fibroids to cervical erosion.

Chest disorders may lead to a loss of blood from coughing, you can lose a lot from a nosebleed, while kidney and bladder disorders may cause blood to appear in the urine. All these different problems can lead to iron deficiency anaemia as a result of the blood loss. Another major cause of deficiency of usable haemoglobin is haemolysis, which, you will recall, is bleeding inside the blood vessels themselves because the skins of the red cells break. The haemoglobin released into the fluid part of the blood, the plasma, is lost to the body as it passes out in the urine. This is called haemoglobinuria (see page 84). There are various causes of haemolysis, including:

- incompatible blood transfusion;
- certain drugs and medicines (see page 31);
- severe burns;
- some snake and spider bites;
- malaria, tuberculosis, liver disease, some hereditary blood disorders (see page 88).

All these things can cause iron deficiency anaemia because loss of haemoglobin means a disproportionate loss of iron, but for 99 per cent of us simple bleeding – for instance because of heavy periods or anti-arthritic medication – is at the root of the problem.

## *Inadequate diet*

If you eat an ordinary mix of foods, you probably take in 15–20mg of iron every day, but you will only absorb about a tenth of this: 1mg daily for a man, a little more for a woman. As you lose about 1mg a day in the skin you shed, this is a tight balance. It seems necessary, therefore, to have much more iron available than you actually retain. In parts of Aberdeenshire and South Wales the amount of iron in the diet is seriously inadequate. This is reflected in very low haemoglobin levels among the people living in these areas. Obviously this is largely a matter of diet: too much oatmeal, bannocks, baps, scones and potato cakes, but not enough meat and fresh greens. The best foods for providing iron include, liver, red meat, sardines and Allbran (see page 24), but you must beware of unrefined cereals. The vitamin C in fresh fruit is also necessary to enable you to absorb the iron.

## Malabsorption

Even when there is iron available, you may not be able to absorb what you need. Phytic acid (see page 96), found in cereals and eggs, prevents the proper absorption of iron. The tannin in tea and alkali medicines (used to treat indigestion), have a similar effect. These substances act by forming an insoluble compound with the iron so that it cannot dissolve in the blood and body fluids. It is like putting a stone into your drink instead of a sugar lump. Vitamin C in large quantities reverses this effect and, surprisingly, white sugar helps. Taking extra iron only helps if you eat a certain amount of meat.

## What is the treatment for iron deficiency anaemia?

### The main treatment

The treatment for this common disease is cheap and easy: you need to take iron tablets. You might think 'the natural way' – changing to a diet rich in iron – would be better. Unfortunately, while a good diet may prevent anaemia, it is too late once you have the disorder. A vicious circle has been set up as the more anaemic you are, the more easily you bleed (for instance, during periods) and the less hearty is your appetite. The most effective compound is the salt, iron sulphate, in a dose of 200mg (which is the normal tablet size), which provides 67mg of pure iron. You need to take one of these tablets three times a day.

This sounds simple enough, but why can't you take it all at once? If you take the iron with or after a meal, you won't absorb it as well as if your stomach were empty, and there is a limit as to how much it can deal with at any one time. The next snag is that once your stomach has received a dose of iron, it refuses to accept any more for about six hours. So, this is why you need to spread the total dosage, taking some on three separate occasions, preferably before meals. Of course, you will also need to avoid phytic-containing wholemeal bread and brown rice and have no more than one egg a week, but go instead for white bread, white sugar and plenty of vitamin C to get the most benefit from the pills.

## The side-effects

All this sounds easy in theory, but a good many people have problems with taking iron, such as stomach pains, diarrhoea, gas or constipation. The slow-release preparations, aimed at bypassing the stomach, are unfortunately less efficacious as the iron is released too far down for it to be absorbed. There are liquid preparations, which are useful for giving to children, and also some chewable tablets containing a small dose of iron for toddlers upwards. Other iron salts are also less upsetting than the sulphate preparations, but they provide only half as much iron, so you need to take them for longer.

The beneficial effects of iron medication begin to show in about two weeks, and your doctor will monitor your progress by checking your blood to see that the haemoglobin level gradually rises. If it doesn't, it is an indication that the underlying cause is still there. When your haemoglobin has reached a normal level, you must continue with the treatment for a further three to six months to replenish your stores.

## Other forms of treatment

### Iron injections

A very few people are unlucky enough to find it impossible to take iron by mouth because of pain, vomiting and diarrhoea or they may have severe anaemia during late pregnancy or after major surgery. For them injections are the only option. The dose is usually given as one injection a day into the muscles, and will be carefully calculated according to your size. Too much is poisonous, and dangerous if it gets into a vein instead of muscle. Equally, small children are in mortal danger if they take adult iron tablets by mouth.

## Blood transfusion

This is an immediate treatment for severe anaemia, but with it comes the risk of a strain being put on the heart in a severely anaemic person.

Transfusions or iron injections or even taking tablets for too long without checking the blood regularly can cause 'iron overload'. This can also occur in alcoholic cirrhosis, heavy drinking of cheap red wine or South African country beer or among the Bantus who do all their cooking for hours and hours in big iron pots. Too much iron causes liver problems, but a little extra does no harm. While it is a mistake to go on taking iron tablets indefinitely (for instance, after you have fully recovered from anaemia of pregnancy), it makes good sense to stick to the preventive diet in the long term (see page 94).

# 6

## Anaemia due to shortage of vitamin $B_{12}$

The Labour Government of 1945, with its landslide majority, lost no time in pushing ahead with a mammoth programme of welfare reform. The pressure on ministers was enormous. Hugh Dalton, the ebullient Chancellor of the Exchequer, needed the constant stimulation of amphetamines – then considered perfectly acceptable – to keep up the pace. He was probably high on Benzedrine in 1947 when he made the disastrous gaffe of revealing a Budget secret to a journalist that brought about his resignation. He was replaced by Stafford Cripps, a model of rectitude, high thoughts and plain living. His puritanical views were so well known that Churchill, gazing across the arid wastes of the Western Desert, had remarked, 'How Cripps would love this.'

With his austere lifestyle, Stafford Cripps was the last man you would expect to show any weakness, so the rest of the group were surprised by his fainting attack on a trip to Simla to see Gandhi. The altitude of the place would have put a strain on the haemoglobin resources of the visitors, but there was no reason to suppose that Cripps was at particular risk, as an anaemic individual would have been. Nor did anyone see any significance in his intractably bad sleep and poor digestion, which was commonplace enough on such a visit. In 1949, when he had been in office less than two years, Cripps' colleagues began to remark on how exhausted he sounded when he was speaking in the House, so he booked himself into a Swiss clinic for six weeks.

The results were gratifying, if startling. He was spotted running round the garden at 5am, completely naked, to the amazement of the staff at the Washington Embassy. Eccentric, if no worse. Then, the pound was devalued and the Finance Bill had a stormy passage. Cripps couldn't cope, so he resigned and returned to the Swiss clinic. Now his main physical problem was back pain, which seemed to have no definite cause. Several months in a plaster cast helped – temporarily. He died in 1952, his illness still a mystery.

Cripps' illness would be no mystery today. It was consistent

52

with Cripps' asceticism – alcohol never passed his lips – that he should be vegetarian. As far back as 1942, Maisky, the Russian Ambassador, was surprised that Cripps only ate a few vegetables at a State banquet. At another prestigious dinner he was noted to confine himself to mashed carrots and orange juice. He had become a vegan. Veganism was fashionable among the intelligentsia at that time, and 'vegan back' was known to affect some of its devotees. Doctors commented on increasing mental symptoms among vegans and a worrying propensity for sudden, unexplained deaths.

It is easy with hindsight and our modern knowledge to trace the clues to Stafford Cripps' illness and suggest what could have cured it. However, it was not until 1948 that cobalamin, vitamin B$_{12}$, was isolated, and several years after that before its vital role in the production of haemoglobin was worked out and anaemia due to vitamin B$_{12}$ deficiency recognized. Vitamin B$_{12}$ is the one vitamin that is not found in any fruit or vegetable. If he had lived a few years later, Cripps could have been saved from his suffering.

Apart from his deadly vegan diet, there was another lethal factor in Cripps' lifestyle. At that time smoking was considered a harmless, even healthy, adjunct to daily life, and Cripps was an exceptionally heavy smoker. He chain-smoked through meetings and conferences and, in the evenings, he continued non-stop: cigarettes, cigars and pipe tobacco in turn. His scant supply of vitamin B$_{12}$ would have been depleted still further by this as tobacco smoke contains cyanide, and the vitamin is used by the body to detoxify it. Most of us, of course, can easily afford to draw on our reserves for this purpose, but not a vegan.

There was one further, apparently innocent, circumstance that contributed to Stafford Cripps' anaemia: a gross imbalance between his intake of vitamin B$_{12}$ and that of folate. These two vitamins act in combination as an essential step in making blood. Vitamin B$_{12}$ is found only in food from animal sources and folate particularly in those from plants. If vitamin B$_{12}$ is in short supply in the body, too much folate is dangerous. It uses up the scanty vitamin B$_{12}$, with especially damaging effects on the nervous system. Cripps' later mental difficulties, his back pain and weakness were no doubt precipitated by his excessive and exclusive intake of fruit, vegetables and nuts: all loaded with folate but devoid of vitamin $B_{12}$.

Poor Stafford Cripps must have had a miserable time. His vague symptoms and those with no physical cause that the doctors could identify would have led to the conviction by colleagues, friends and the professionals that his problems were 'all in the mind'. This type of misinterpretation can still happen today, but at least we know about vitamin $B_{12}$ and vitamin $B_{12}$ deficiency anaemia, and how to put it right.

The first essential, even now, is to take note of any warnings. Even if you are starting to lack vitamin $B_{12}$, you won't have all the possible symptoms. The trick is to be alert to any you do have and, if they persist over several weeks, get them checked out.

## *The signs and symptoms of vitamin $B_{12}$ deficiency*

These are as follows.

- Any of the general symptoms of anaemia (see pages 18–19). As with all forms of anaemia, some of its effects, such as the poor sleep and easy fatigue suffered by Stafford Cripps, may be passed off as due to worry, the weather, your age or any of a host of other reasons.
- A beefy-red, sore tongue – often the first sign of the illness. It is worse with hot foods or those with sharp flavours. The inflammation comes and goes, regardless of what you do.
- Alternatively, the tongue may be smooth and pale.
- Soreness and cracks at the corners of the mouth, though these are far less common than they are in iron deficiency anaemia.
- Pale skin and mucous membranes, which, as the anaemia becomes more severe, take on a lemony tint, including the whites of the eyes. This is because the red blood cells cannot develop properly and tend to leak their haemoglobin into the plasma. There its red colour changes to yellow. You may not notice the change in your appearance yourself – a friend you haven't seen for ages or a new doctor may be the first to draw your attention to it.
- Darkening of the urine is an occasional secondary effect.

- In a few cases, the skin darkens quite a lot with the natural pigment melanin. No one knows the reason for this.
- Bruises appear mysteriously, often on your thighs or arms, although you have not knocked them.
- You have diarrhoea out of the blue from time to time, bearing no relation to what you have been eating.
- The changes in your blood may lead to clotting in a vein or blockage in an artery with local symptoms that are sure to take you to the doctor, such as swelling, pain, redness and heat.
- Heart problems. If the anaemia has crept up on you so gradually that you have not noticed anything untoward, the first indication of trouble may be the beginnings of heart failure, of the slow, congestive type. You are short of breath with any effort, and your ankles may swell; you have no energy.
- Infertility – a possibility to bear in mind if there is no more obvious cause for it.
- Possible serious effects on your unborn child if you are short of vitamin B$_{12}$ during pregnancy. However, vitamin B$_{12}$ deficiency in pregnancy is very rare in the West as it only crops up as a result of dire poverty, such as there is in some developing countries, or when the mother is eating a really weird diet, such as eating only one kind of food to the exclusion of all others or a very restricted range of foods. The worst ill effect is spina bifida, but cleft lip or palate may also result.
- An unexpected inability to throw off an infection may be the first you know of a slowly developing, but severe, lack of vitamin B$_{12}$. The blood-making arrangements in your bone marrow are thrown so out of kilter by this lack that they cannot produce the components of the body's defence system.

A large group of symptoms involving the nervous system and brain affect some people.

- Pins and needles, burning or tingling, or numbness and cold, usually starting in your feet first and later your hands. These sensations affect both sides equally and they usher in the nervous symptoms of the illness in 80 per cent of cases. It may not click in your doctor's mind that this could be caused by a vitamin deficiency syndrome.

- 'Glove and stocking anaesthesia', which means a loss of sensation in your hands and feet. You may lose your joint sense too, which makes controlling your legs especially difficult.
- Difficulty in keeping your balance when you walk, so that you easily trip and fall.
- Muscular weakness and stiffness, also most troublesome in your legs. You tend to drag your toes as you walk.
- Blurring of vision as the optic nerve – the one that serves your eyesight – may be damaged by lack of vitamin B$_{12}$.
- Muddled thinking, forgetfulness, lack of usual interest and initiative. This can shade into dementia over time, if not corrected.

The symptoms of vitamin B$_{12}$ deficiency showing up in the nervous system only occur in a minority of people, but together are called, rather alarmingly, subacute combined degeneration of the cord. The 'cord' referred to is the spinal cord, that column of nerves running down inside your backbone, connecting with the nerves to the limbs and brain. Sometimes the nervous system reacts to a lack of vitamin B$_{12}$ without there also being anaemia, but the cause and the cure are the same in either case.

While pins and needles are most often the first symptom of the complex, any of the others may be, including the fall-off in intellectual ability. This last may not be recognized until the victim begins to recover. Then, as the mental alertness comes back with treatment, it becomes clear that the person had not been himself mentally for many months. The victims are nearly always elderly, and more often men. Nevertheless, neither sex, nor any age, is immune. Judith, for example, was only 33 when she began to lose her intellectual edge in her high-powered sales job. She made a complete recovery.

*Alan*

Alan was typical. He was 73 and had been right through World War II in the tank corps, as he liked to tell his passengers, and he hadn't had a day's illness, except for a bit of trouble with his bowels now and then. Alan fell into low spirits when he was told he must give up his work as a London cabby. At his age you have to have a medical every year and this time his eyesight did not pass the test.

After that he seemed to go downhill. He became increasingly forgetful – he who had prided himself on his grasp of the Knowledge – and he lost all his get-up-and-go. He couldn't even rouse himself to follow the football. Also, his walking was definitely unsteady and he had had one or two nasty falls. They shake you up when you are over 70, but neither his family nor Alan himself thought it was out of the way for a man of his age to be a trifle vague and to stumble occasionally. A case of anno domini, the GP had said reassuringly, and advised Alan to 'take it easy'. After all, he was well past retirement age.

It was a locum, filling in while Alan's usual doctor was on holiday, who decided to look into the possibilities and see if anything could be done to perk him up. He looked on Alan's symptoms with a fresh eye, unlike Alan's own GP who was lulled by his familiarity with him into thinking that Alan seemed much as he always did, only a little older. Alan's blood tests showed that he was severely anaemic and that his serum B$_{12}$ was alarmingly low. The injections worked a miracle.

In Alan's case it had not been a matter of a poor diet – his wife saw to it that he ate well – but his bowel problem that had led to his anaemia.

## The causes of vitamin B$_{12}$ deficiency

The causes are the following.

- A vegan or other diet deficient in animal products.
- An excess of folate, as a result of taking very large doses of folic acid tablets or following the same sort of diet and lifestyle as Stafford Cripps, as excess of folate in food can tip the balance by using up an already scanty supply of vitamin B$_{12}$.
- Overgrowth of bacteria in the intestines. This can occur in diverticular disease, which is when a wear and tear effect causes little pouches to develop in which the normally harmless germs

present there can multiply. This may cause loose bowels and discomfort, but these symptoms may be very slight. The snag is that the bacteria prevent the intestine from absorbing the usual amount of vitamin B$_{12}$, as happened to Alan. Treatment with tetracycline damps down the infection.

- Crohn's disease (a serious problem affecting the small intestines more than the colon) also impairs absorption of vitamin B$_{12}$. Sometimes it causes a fistula, or passageway, to form, joining two loops of gut and bypassing a section, which then becomes a breeding ground for germs.

- Coeliac disease usually appears before the age of two, but occasionally it is not recognized until adult life. It is a congenital lack of the enzymes that enable us to absorb gluten, which is in ordinary foodstuffs, such as wheat products. Vitamin B$_{12}$ is poorly absorbed, too. The children who are affected are obviously unable to thrive, while adults who have it are slightly anaemic and vaguely ill.

- Stomach operations or chronic gastritis also disturb absorption. They, thus, often lead to pernicious anaemia.

- Some parasites, for instance the fish tapeworm, which is present in raw fish dishes, can use up all the available vitamin B$_{12}$. Meat from fish-eating animals in Scandinavia and Asia can also introduce the tapeworm. Effective medicines are niclosomide or praziquantil, while thoroughly cooking fish or meat is the preventive.

- Diabetic diarrhoea may occur because diabetes sometimes upsets the nerves controlling the muscles of the intestines, resulting in constipation or watery diarrhoea, typically in the night. In this situation, vitamin B$_{12}$ cannot be absorbed and anaemia develops.

- Stagnant loop syndrome. Your 6.7m (22ft) of intestines lie in closely packed coils and loops in your abdomen and, generally, so long as the partly digested food travels down them at a steady rate, squeezed along by the intestinal muscles, no problems arise. There are always bacteria in the gut, which play an essential role in breaking down the food for digestion and absorption. The muscular movement can become sluggish under the influence of several types of medicine, including painkillers, tranquillizers, sleeping tablets and antidepressants, and a general slow-down occurs as we get older. In these circumstances, a loop of gut may be missed out by the general flow – a so-called stagnant or blind loop – and then a build-up of material can occur where bacteria will multiply, sometimes up to two or three times their normal numbers. This results in bouts of colicky pain and loose motions, which may be pale and fatty or sometimes dark with blood. Obviously then the intestine cannot do its work of absorbing all the proteins, fats, carbohydrates and vitamin B$_{12}$ needed. Two special types of X-ray are used to confirm the diagnosis of this problem: a barium swallow and a barium enema. These involve taking in, by mouth or anus, a liquid containing barium, which is used because it shows up on the X-ray film and gives a picture of any abnormality in the gut. If there is some anatomical quirk at the root of the problem, this will need to be remedied surgically, but more often tetracycline is given to control the excess of bacteria. The dosage is 1–2g daily and it is effective within three to four days and then the vitamin B$_{12}$ and other nutrients will start to be absorbed properly once more. If the underlying condition is likely to continue, a seven- to ten-day long course of tetracycline should be taken every six months, indefinitely.

### *Medicines that interfere with the absorption of vitamin B$_{12}$*
These are:

- neomycin, an antifungal used in the treatment of some skin and ear problems;
- metformin (Glucophage), used to treat diabetes.

## Special tests

Blood tests can be done to see if there is:

- a very low haemoglobin level;
- a reduced number of red cells.

A chemical test will register whether or not the:

- serum vitamin B$_{12}$ level is reduced.

A blood film viewed under the microscope will show up:

- oversized red cells;
- oddly shaped red cells.

Other screening tests that are done to check if there are other causes of this blood picture are:

- liver function;
- thyroid function;
- Schilling test (see page 67).

These three tests give normal results if the problem is purely a lack of vitamin B$_{12}$.

## What is the treatment for vitamin B$_{12}$ deficiency?

### In an emergency

If your haemoglobin level is very low (less than 4g/dl), you will need a blood transfusion. This should preferably be in the form of a concentrate of red blood cells, given slowly so as not to put a strain on the heart by suddenly expecting it to pump round an extra quantity of blood. Frusemide (a water tablet) is given for the same reason (to reduce the volume of fluid in the body).

### The standard treatment

This consists of injections of hydroxocobalamin (vitamin B$_{12}$), each of 1000mg. These are given twice a day for a week, once a week for the next six weeks and, after that, four times a year for life. If your vitamin B$_{12}$ anaemia resulted solely from your being a vegan and you alter your diet, an injection just once a year should keep you topped up.

The bone marrow swings into full production within 48 hours of the first dose of vitamin B$_{12}$ being given and normal, healthy red cells begin flooding your bloodstream days after that. All this production of haemoglobin-filled red cells may use up your reserves of iron, though, so your doctor may also prescribe a course of iron tablets, starting soon after the injections have begun. Your blood film will show extra pale red cells when you are short of iron.

## Helen

Helen was 59, warm-hearted and comfortably plump. Her three grandchildren loved visiting her. One of the high spots of their visits was tea, with the scrumptious cakes and biscuits she made, decorated with sweets.

Her diabetes was a nuisance, but she did not let it spoil everything. It had developed about four years ago, just after Jim had had his coronary. The doctor said it was the mature-onset type of diabetes and quite mild, so she should be able to control it by means of diet alone. This very quickly proved to be impossible.

It wasn't that Helen ate a lot, but she liked the wrong things: cakes, scones, cornflakes and, of course, vegetables, including potatoes (chips were her favourite), as well as the apple a day that was supposed to keep the doctor away. She wasn't a great one for meat, especially since Jim died – it didn't seem worth cooking just for her. Her new dentures did not help either.

In the end the doctor said she had better have some antidiabetic tablets, so he started her on Glucophage. With these, and doing the best she could about her diet, Helen's diabetes came under reasonable control. Of course, she had to continue with the tablets, but she wasn't aware of any side-effects.

All that had happened several years before. Lately, Helen had been feeling increasingly tired and listless – partly, perhaps because she'd had a run of minor infections. It was only a small thing, but her feet were like blocks of ice and her fingers often went dead, even when it wasn't particularly cold. Then there was that big purple bruise that had appeared as if by magic – she certainly couldn't remember bumping herself. What was more troublesome, though, was getting so puffed at the slightest exertion, and sometimes feeling slightly nauseous.

When she went for her next routine visit to have her diabetes checked, Helen mentioned how she was getting short of breath and feeling generally under par. The doctor gave her a thorough examination, including an electrocardiogram (to check her heart) and a blood test.

Helen was found to be severely anaemic, and it was putting a strain on her heart as it was having to pump the poor-quality blood round at an increased rate to supply her organs with sufficient oxygen. Her anaemia was of the sort caused by a shortage of vitamin B$_{12}$. Her diet was not ideal, but the basic cause of Helen's anaemia was the Glucophage, one of the drugs that may, in some people, prevent the body from using the vitamin B$_{12}$ in their food. Helen's store of this vitamin meant that it took two or three years for the deficiency to manifest itself.

Helen took a long time to recover completely, but with rest, heart tablets, vitamin B$_{12}$ injections and, later, some iron tablets, she did get better. The Glucophage – the culprit – was replaced with a different antidiabetic tablet and, for the sake of her heart as well as her diabetes, Helen has managed to reduce her weight.

There are other important causes of anaemia that results in outsized red blood corpuscles:

- pernicious anaemia (see Chapter 7);
- folate (folic acid) deficiency (see Chapter 8).

# 7

## Pernicious anaemia, or Addisonian anaemia

Pernicious anaemia is a particular form of anaemia that results from a deficiency of vitamin $B_{12}$. It is more common than any of the other kinds, accounting for about 80 per cent of sufferers. Until the middle of the twentieth century, it was invariably fatal, but thankfully, we know how to treat it now. It is also more mysterious than the other kinds of anaemia as it is not due to any shortage of vitamin $B_{12}$ in the diet, nor to malabsorption.

In 1849, Dr Thomas Addison of Guy's Hospital in London first described a group of his patients with this illness. It had nothing to do with a lack of iron – the only known cause of anaemia at that time – and all the victims died. It was feared as much as cancer is today. Although the disease was named after him and he was desperate to help the victims, Dr Addison could find no cure.

The breakthrough did not come until 1926. Two Americans, Doctors Minot and Murphy from Massachusetts, found that eating large quantities of raw liver every day would keep their pernicious anaemia patients alive and well. We know now that this was because of the vitamin $B_{12}$ stored in liver, but no one had even heard of this vitamin until after World War II.

A Dr William Castle went to a lecture by Dr Minot and came away intrigued. There was obviously something in liver that the anaemic patients needed. He called this the 'extrinsic factor', as it came from outside the body, but as ordinary people don't need vast quantities of liver to stay fit, he reckoned that there was something lacking in the anaemic patients themselves. He called this the 'intrinsic factor'. He tracked it down to the gastric juice – the digestive juice produced in the stomach. Even when they were topped up with liver and apparently well, Dr Castle found that his patients' gastric juice was different from healthy people's, but 70 years ago there was not the technology to analyse it.

Dr Castle found that if he brought up his own healthy stomach contents, there was something in them that made his pernicious anaemia patients feel much better without all that liver. Presumably he did not spell out to them where he had obtained the 'new medicine'. As he could not provide an ongoing supply, the patients had to continue taking liver, but at least their illness was now better understood and they survived. In due course, concentrated liver extract was manufactured and then produced in an injectable form, so the treatment was not so unpleasant.

The second breakthrough came in 1948 when, simultaneously in Britain and America, vitamin $B_{12}$, or cobalamin, was isolated, and, a few years later, was available as an injection. No one today dies of pernicious anaemia, nor need they even feel poorly because of it.

## How does pernicious anaemia come about?

The underlying cause of pernicious anaemia is a lack of usable vitamin $B_{12}$ in the body. This, as we have seen, is because of the absence of intrinsic factor in the gastric juices. This, in turn, comes about because of an autoimmune reaction.

Pernicious anaemia is one of a group of autoimmune diseases in which the body's defence system turns against some of its own cells – in this case, the gastric parietal cells. If any of your blood relatives has one of the autoimmune disorders, you are more likely than most to get one or more of them yourself.

Another autoimmune disease that very often occurs in those with pernicious anaemia is vitiligo, and as it affects the skin it is easy to spot. The skin is perfectly smooth and healthy and feels no different from usual, but it loses its brown pigment, melanin, in patches, which show up as they are moderately or completely white. They can occur anywhere on the face and body and the condition gradually spreads. It seems worse in the summer because, as the rest of the skin tans in the sun, the areas of vitiligo remain obstinately pale. Make-up is a useful measure to cover patches on the face.

## Special characteristics of pernicious anaemia

These are as follows.

- It can affect people of any race, anywhere, but is rare in the tropics and especially common in Northern Europe. Even so it

64

affects only 1 in 10,000 people.
- Blue-eyed people are more likely to be affected than those with brown eyes.
- There is a tendency to go grey prematurely.
- Women more often affected than men, in the ratio of 3 to 2.
- It is unusual for it to occur in those under 30, and is likeliest in women of 45 to 65, peaking at the age of 60.
- It has a preference for those with blood group A blood, which accounts for 41 per cent of people in Britain.
- Other autoimmune disorders likely to crop up in those with pernicious anaemia or their relatives include:
  - vitiligo (see above);
  - diabetes;
  - rheumatoid arthritis;
  - underactive thyroid (Hashimoto type);
  - overactive thyroid;
  - systemic lupus erythematosus (SLE);
  - some liver diseases;
  - dermatomyositis.

## Signs and symptoms to look out for

These all result from a deficiency of usable vitamin $B_{12}$, and are listed in full in the previous chapter, pages 54–6, and you may also have some of the general symptoms of all kinds of anaemia, on pages 18–19.

Look out for:

- pallor, with a faint lemon yellow tint, including the whites of your eyes;
- occasionally, a darkening of the skin all over, but especially noticeable in the skin folds;
- a pale and smooth tongue or sometimes sore, red and inflamed;
- pins and needles in your feet and hands;
- loss of weight, but you don't look as though you've lost any;
- memory and concentration difficulties, or almost any psychological symptoms – from panics to mild dementia;

- deadly fatigue, as in all types of anaemia, but likely to be particularly severe with this form as it is apt to be well advanced before the illness is recognized;
- tendency to bleed unduly, for instance having heavy periods, nosebleeds and so on (this is a sign that the blood production process going on in the bone marrow is so desperately short of vitamin $B_{12}$ that the blood platelets, which aid clotting, are not being produced in adequate numbers).

Pernicious anaemia is an illness that creeps up on you slowly and gently, with symptoms and signs that don't ring immediate alarm bells and so you may not realize the urgency of the need for treatment. However, if it is not treated, you are on a one-way trip to disaster, with the loss of physical health, your sanity and, finally, your life.

## The investigations that may be done when pernicious anaemia is suspected

The following tests and the results listed would indicate that you have this form of anaemia:

- blood film when outsized red corpuscles that are oval instead of round and some odd shapes would be seen;
- a haemoglobin check would show it to be at a low or very low level;
- a red cell count would produce low numbers;
- a serum iron check would reveal it to be at a high level;
- a serum vitamin $B_{12}$ check would show it to be at a very low level.

### Test results which are only positive in cases of pernicious anaemia

The following results would confirm a diagnosis of this illness:

- presence of anti-intrinsic factor antibodies in the blood (in up to 50 per cent of cases);

- lack of normal stomach acid;
- abnormal Schilling test, which is when a dose of vitamin $B_{12}$ given by mouth is not properly absorbed unless intrinsic factor is given as well (in ordinary vitamin $B_{12}$ deficiency, adding the intrinsic factor makes no difference as it is absorbed anyway).

## *Edith*

She had been a glamorous girl at 19 – a blue-eyed honey blonde – and her appearance was just as important to her at 69.

She was of the generation before suntan became fashionable and so kept out of the sun. As she was proud of her pale skin, she did not mind that it seemed to be getting even paler. She explained away the yellowish tinge with something she'd read about blondes having green undertones to their complexion. If green, why not yellow? On the other hand, she had been disappointed when her hair had lost every vestige of colour by the time she was 50. Now, heading towards 70, it looked elegant to have snowy white hair.

Then the vitiligo started. Patches of really white skin appeared and spread, making the remaining pale skin look unattractively muddy and yellowish by comparison. The notion of leprosy came to Edith's mind, but the doctor assured her that it was perfectly harmless. He was, as usual, busy and was glad when Edith told him that otherwise she was quite well. She had been fortunate with her health for most of her life, although she was sad to have had no children. She and John had certainly tried.

It was Edith's legs that let her down. She'd had the odd tingling sensations in her feet for years, but now she found her walking rather unsteady. Particularly when it was dark, she liked to find a rail to hang on to. When the practice that Edith's GP belonged to wrote and offered all its senior patients a thorough check-up she decided to go along. Ordinarily she did not like to bother her doctor. He might think she was fussing about nothing if she complained about such things as feeling tired, not sleeping too well and forgetting what she had done with her key, but this was an open invitation to do so.

The nurse carrying out the screening was worried when she saw Edith and asked the doctor to have a look at her. After he had examined her, he told her that she was anaemic and arranged some tests.

These showed that Edith had a very low haemoglobin level (6g/dl), big oval red cells, and she had a positive Schilling test. She had severe pernicious anaemia and she needed to receive treatment urgently.

It must have been coming on for years, the doctor said, to have got so bad; it might even have been involved in her inability to have a baby. Sadly, that had been a factor in her divorce.

When the doctor asked her whether or not there were autoimmune illnesses in the family, Edith remembered an aunt, years ago, who had a thyroid problem and might have been anaemic, too, but, of course, Edith had not thought this to be relevant to her own health.

The specialist her doctor had brought in decided that, as her haemoglobin level was very low, Edith should start her treatment with a blood transfusion. The effect of this was immediate. She felt as though life itself had been introduced into her veins, and when this was followed by the first few weeks of vitamin $B_{12}$ injections Edith felt – and looked – ten years younger and stronger and happier.

## Look-alike anaemia

If, for an ulcer or some other stomach problem, you have to have part of it removed, you run a 50 per cent risk of developing a syndrome that is just like pernicious anaemia, with a shortage of vitamin $B_{12}$ and intrinsic factor. This is because the cells lining the stomach, which make the intrinsic factor, and the stomach acid have been removed.

There is also a lesser procedure called vagotomy in which a nerve to the stomach is cut deliberately to switch off the production of acid. The snag with this is that it also stops the production of intrinsic factor.

The treatment for these look-alike cases of anaemia is the same as for pernicious anaemia.

## What is the treatment for pernicious anaemia?

A blood transfusion is a life-saver in any case of very severe anaemia (see page 20).

Injections of hydroxocobalamin (vitamin $B_{12}$), each injection being of 1000mg into a big muscle:

- twice in the first week, then;
- once a week for six weeks, then;
- two to four times a year (with tests to assess your progress) for the rest of your life.

### How do the injections work?

Ordinarily, vitamin $B_{12}$ and the extrinsic factor, which is in some of your food (for instance, meat), comes into contact with the intrinsic factor in your stomach. The two factors are made for each other and immediately join together. The combination travels a long way down the small intestine until it reaches a special place, just before the colon or large intestine begins. There the two factors uncouple and the vitamin is absorbed into the bloodstream to be used, and the intrinsic factor is discarded along with the other waste products. The two factors combine temporarily in this way to save the vitamin $B_{12}$ from being digested with the rest of the food until it reaches the safe area at the end of the small intestine. If you have no intrinsic factor (because of autoimmune antibodies or surgery), it is useless to give you vitamin $B_{12}$ by mouth because it will be destroyed by the digestive juices. The injections, however, bypass that difficulty.

An injection two or three times a year is a small price to pay for normal health and far better than the alternative – 225g ($\frac{1}{2}$lb) of raw liver every single day!

The playwright, George Bernard Shaw, suffered from pernicious anaemia and, to make matters worse, he was a committed vegetarian. He would sneer at people who ate meat, saying that the amount of goodness in a steak was as nothing compared with that of an acorn, as the latter could grow into a great oak tree. There is no record of what he said when his doctors insisted that the only treatment for his condition was raw liver, and then concentrated liver extract.

# 8

# Folate (or folic acid) deficiency and aplastic anaemias

By the 1930s, doctors knew about the commonest form of anaemia due to lack of iron, and the far more dangerous pernicious anaemia that could be kept in check by something in raw liver, which we now know to be vitamin $B_{12}$.

Dr Lucy Wills, a pioneering doctor working in Bombay in 1931, was distressed at the number of pregnant women who became ill. They were generally poorly and exhausted, and instead of gaining weight, they tended to lose it – a worrying situation in pregnancy. These mothers were anaemic, and they very often died when their babies were born because of the inevitable loss of blood during the birth. Iron tonics did not help them and, anyway, their symptoms – for instance, pins and needles or an inflamed tongue – were more reminiscent of pernicious than iron deficiency anaemia. Also, under the microscope, they had big, oval red cells, not the little round ones that occur in iron deficiency. Eating liver did not help, so Dr Wills guessed that there must be something else they were lacking.

She considered their diet, which consisted mainly of rice or bread with very little meat or vegetables. So she tried giving the same food to monkeys, and they, too, became weak and weary like the women. After running through all the foods she could think of, Dr Wills hit on one that cured the problem: yeast extract (Marmite). She still did not know about folate, or folic acid, as this vitamin had yet to be discovered, but this was the factor in the yeast extract that cured her patients.

Folate works in conjunction with vitamin $B_{12}$ to enable the body to make DNA, which, as we have seen, is the essential blueprint for the production of all new cells. As red blood cells have a strictly limited life, as well as being the most numerous of all the cells in the body, anything that inhibits cell production affects them most. It leads to a type of anaemia in which there is a reduced number of red cells and many of the ones remaining are of the wrong size and shape. A shortage either of vitamin $B_{12}$ or of folate produces these

71

effects, and the symptoms and signs and the appearance of the blood when it is examined under a microscope are similar in both cases.

## What are the causes of lack of folate?

### Diet

Folate is found in some meats and, to a lesser extent, in raw vegetables.

A diet based on bread, rice or pasta or overcooked food is likely to be short in folate. Vegetarians, including strict vegans, Hindus and the Indian populations of South Africa and Fiji, are all at high risk of folate deficiency anaemia.

Babies fed exclusively on goat's milk will also be short of folate, whereas in human or cow's milk there is just enough of this vitamin for their needs.

In Britain, America and other Western countries, the only people likely to have a diet deficient in folate are the old, poor and housebound, existing on bread, buns and biscuits, with a little porridge and milk, or those following extreme diets for other reasons. A diet low in or lacking folate (for instance when you are ill) will have an effect on your blood within days.

### Pregnancy

The developing baby uses up vast amounts of its mother's reserves of vitamin $B_{12}$ and folate. Although her store of vitamin $B_{12}$ is ample to see her through pregnancy and the period around the time of the birth, the folate store is quickly used up.

Many mothers feel nauseous and eat very little, especially meat and vegetables, in the first 12 weeks of pregnancy, yet these are vital weeks in the baby's development. In fact, to avoid all possible danger of spina bifida or other serious congenital disorders of the nervous system, women are advised to start taking supplements of folic acid as soon as they are even planning to conceive! Often women only start to take supplements once they know they are pregnant, but this is adequate.

It is not only in early pregnancy that folate is important. In the last half the baby is growing so fast that it needs a big, steady supply of folate, and everything else (see page 4).

## Physical illness

Any illness, especially if there is inflammation, calls for extra supplies of folate, which is required by the body so that it can repair itself. Examples are TB, malaria, skin diseases such as eczema, dermatitis with peeling, Crohn's disease of the intestine, and all forms of liver disorder. Interestingly, in stagnant loop syndrome, which, you will recall, is a cause of vitamin $B_{12}$ deficiency (page 58), there is actually an increase in folate levels as the bacteria trapped in the blind loop can manufacture folate.

## Coeliac disease

This is a particularly important disease in terms of its effect on folate metabolism. Indeed, it is always associated with a lack of folate. Coeliac disease involves an inability to digest gluten, a component of wheat, and, secondarily, the absorption of folate is reduced. This may take a year or more to show.

Coeliac disease usually arises before the age of two. The child with this disease will be obviously ill and the doctor will be involved. If the illness, including a lack of folate, develops later in childhood, the youngster's growth is held back and puberty delayed. In other cases, however, the syndrome is not diagnosed until adult life, although it is likely to have been present for some years, but with symptoms too mild to arouse concern. The usual symptoms are diarrhoea, loss of weight and anaemia, but in some elderly patients there is no diarrhoea.

## Natasha

Natasha was 16 and only 1.2m (4ft 8in) tall when her mother started to worry seriously. Her daughter seemed to be a girl Peter Pan – her body was still a sexless child shape, with only the tiniest breast buds and almost no pubic hair. She had not started her periods either. The final trigger that made Natasha agree to see the doctor was the soreness and blistering that broke out on her forearms. The doctor said it looked like dermatitis herpetiformis, which is fairly common in coeliac disease, so he asked a few pertinent questions. Natasha did not suffer from diarrhoea, but she was a fussy eater. Although she was underweight, her abdomen bulged out more than you'd expect. She was very pale and generally under par. Investigations by a specialist confirmed her doctor's provisional diagnosis, which was coeliac disease with profound folate deficiency anaemia.

Treatment of the coeliac disease and supplements of folic acid helped Natasha to grow and develop, although she never quite caught up in height. However, the dermatitis faded within a few weeks.

## Kidney disease

Particularly if the person is on haemodialysis, the folate tends to be washed out of the body in the urine. The situation is a little better for those receiving peritoneal dialysis, but folate (folic acid) tablets must be taken.

## Heart disorders

The congestive type of heart trouble makes the liver congested also, and this in turn leads to a loss of folate in the urine.

## Hypothyroidism (an underactive thyroid)

This can be a direct cause of folate deficiency.

## Haemolytic anaemias

Those in which the red blood cells are destroyed, as in sickle cell anaemia, can lead to a shortage of folate among other vital constituents for making blood.

## Alcohol drunk in excess

If this is drunk regularly in substantial quantities, it is a potent cause of folate deficiency and, sometimes, iron deficiency. Around 50 per cent of heavy drinkers are anaemic, although they may be unaware that they are. Spirits are especially harmful, while beer has the redeeming feature of containing folate.

The reasons heavy drinkers have folate deficiency include the following:

74

- the direct toxic effect of alcohol on the bone marrow, interfering with the body's ability to make blood;
- a chronic loss of blood from the digestive tract, which is liable to become inflamed and to ulcerate anywhere along its length, from the oesophagus (gullet) to the anus;
- a tendency to bleed is part of the alcoholic syndrome, especially in people with cirrhosis;
- any liver disorder prevents it dealing properly with vitamin $B_{12}$ and folate as it allows supplies of vitamin $B_{12}$ to build up, but the folate is washed out with the waste;
- anyone on a junk food diet or any other that doesn't provide enough folate will begin to show signs of folate deficiency anaemia within about 19 weeks, but if alcohol is added to the diet, the deficiency shows up within 2 weeks.

*Kirsty*

She came from Scotland, which perhaps accounted for her preference for drinking whisky rather than, say, wine.

She worked in the highly stressful world of advertising and, at 33, had an income that paid for a flat in Chelsea and a silver Mercedes.

Kirsty's very heavy periods, which were getting worse, didn't fit the image, but the symptom that finally sent her to the doctor was the rash. Apart from her propensity for big bruises – 'You've only to look at me and I get a bruise,' she complained – she had a crop of small, flat spots all over her body and limbs. They started off bright red and then changed to purple, finally fading to a brownish-yellow, and then a new lot would appear. Her GP said this was called purpura and that it wasn't an illness, but a reaction. He enquired into her general health.

Kirsty had to admit that she had lost energy and ability to concentrate lately, and even her social life was suffering. Also, although she felt tired, she couldn't sleep and even an alcoholic nightcap didn't help.

Tests showed that Kirsty was anaemic, with big red cells and a shortage of platelets in her blood and a deficiency of folate in the serum.

The cause of her folate deficiency was tracked down to her alcohol intake, as she was trying to keep pace with the men. Treatment to boost her folate level would be useless unless she called a halt to her drinking for several months and, then, if she did return to it her intake would have to be on a very moderate scale. Also, wine would be better for her than whisky, if she were to have alcohol at all.

The good news is that, in most cases of alcohol-induced folate deficiency, there are signs of recovery within a few days of stopping drinking. In particular, the lack of platelets is speedily reversed. This is good because, as you will recall, the platelets are the tiny blood cells that are essential in enabling the blood to clot. Especially in cirrhosis or an acute liver upset, the platelet count plummets and so haemorrhages, small or large, result.

A further disadvantage of alcohol is that it makes antifolate drug reactions more likely. The diuretic (water tablet) triamterene, which normally causes no trouble, has this effect when alcohol is consumed as well. The inhibitory effect on folate of some other drugs is also made worse by alcohol (see below).

## Antifolate drugs

Some medicines can prevent the body from taking up folate, although this doesn't always happen. They include:

- anti-epileptics, such as phenytoin, phenobarbitone and primo-done, which cause folate depletion so often that supplements of the vitamin are given routinely when these are prescibed;
- trimethoprim (Septrim, Bactrim), an antibiotic, which is most likely to cause trouble when it is taken in the long term as a preventive, for instance in the treatment of recurrent bladder infections;
- sulphasalazine, used to treat diseases of the intestines, for instance Crohn's disease, which in itself leads to folate and vitamin $B_{12}$ deficiency;
- pyrimethamine (Daraprim), an anti-malarial;
- triamterene, a diuretic (see above).

## What are the signs and symptoms to look out for?

Folate deficiency anaemia reveals itself in similar ways to those given for vitamin $B_{12}$ deficiency and pernicious anaemia, on pages 54–6 and 65–6, respectively, plus, of course, there are the general symptoms of anaemia, given on pages 18–19. Here are a few of them:

- an inescapable feeling of lassitude;
- pale skin, lips and eyelids, sometimes tinged with lemon;
- shortness of breath on exertion;
- palpitations;
- dizziness;
- your thoughts and ideas are less clearly focused than usual;
- sore tongue;
- occasional diarrhoea;
- mild fever at times;
- tendency to lose weight.

In folate deficiency anaemia the sufferers are likely to be much younger than those with pernicious anaemia or simple $B_{12}$ deficiency. On the whole the symptoms are less severe, and only a minority have a sore red tongue.

## Tests that may be performed when folate deficiency anaemia is suspected

These may include the following, the results given here indicating that this will be the diagnosis:

- a serum folate check, the level being low;
- a red blood corpuscle folate check, with a low level being found;
- a serum vitamin $B_{12}$ check, with a normal or, perhaps, high level of this vitamin;
- an assessment of dietary folate intake;
- a biopsy of the duodenum, to check for coeliac disease;
- a blood film, big, oval cells and some misshapen ones, as in vitamin $B_{12}$ deficiency, showing up under the microscope.

# What is the treatment for this sort of anaemia?

Unlike when there is a deficiency of vitamin $B_{12}$, including pernicious anaemia, which involves you having to have vitamin $B_{12}$ injections for life, you can absorb folate from tablets taken by mouth, and some doctors even suggest that a change of diet alone might cure the problem. However, most people want to get better as soon as possible, and the tablets achieve this.

There is one constraint. If there is an excess of folate in comparison with vitamin $B_{12}$ in the body, the folate can use up the vitamin $B_{12}$ to such an extent that serious neurological and mental problems are likely to develop. Except in pregnancy, when vitamin $B_{12}$ is usually in ample supply (and, anyway, may be checked), it is essential to test the level of vitamin $B_{12}$ in the serum and make sure that it is not depleted before starting folate treatment. A booster vitamin $B_{12}$ injection can be given if necessary.

The usual regime consists of taking one tablet containing 5mg of folic acid daily for four months. It is only necessary to continue after this time if the underlying cause of the lack of folate has not been found and dealt with. In severe sickle cell or other haemolytic anaemia (see Chapter 9), taking one 5mg tablet weekly is a precaution against the folate level dipping down too far. In the forms of haemolytic anaemia, so much new blood is required to make up for what is being lost that you can run short of folate, and other ingredients. As well as the tablets, and continuing with these afterwards, following a diet rich in folate makes good sense. Such a diet includes salads and raw vegetables wherever possible (having them grated helps) and some meat, preferably beef.

# Preventing folate deficiency during pregnancy

Taking the following steps will help to ensure that adequate levels of folate are maintained throughout pregnancy:

- daily doses of 400muG of folic acid (note that larger doses might lead to a relative lack of vitamin $B_{12}$ and symptoms in the nervous system or brain);
- because some serious abnormalities can develop in the unborn

baby in the early days of pregnancy and these can be prevented by the mother's taking folic acid, this should be started as soon as practicable – ideally at the 'twinkle in the eye' stage, when you are actively trying to conceive, but otherwise as early as possible;

- in 1996, the US Food and Drugs Administration required that folic acid should be added to most bread, flour, cornmeal, rice, noodles and macaroni, largely for the sake of mothers and their babies, so eating these foods will provide you with some folic acid;
- a mother who has previously had a baby with an abnormality of the nervous system should take a larger dose of folic acid (5mg) daily as soon as she is contemplating another pregnancy;
- because there is a tendency for mothers-to-be to run short of iron, most folate tablets also contain iron (such as Pregaday and Ferfolic SV), but if there are any side-effects from the combined tablets, such as stomach pain and either constipation or diarrhoea, this will be due to the iron and taking a folic acid-only tablet will avoid these problems.

Premature babies may be given folic acid as a syrup (such as Lexpec) as they are likelier than most babies to be short of this vitamin.

## *What foods provide us with folate?*

Excellent sources are:

- liver, 300muG per 100g;
- raw oysters, 250muG per 100g;
- uncooked spinach, 80muG per 100g;
- uncooked broccoli, 30muG per 100g;
- uncooked cabbage, 20muG per 100g;
- lettuce, 20muG per 100g (but you need a lot of salad to make 100g);
- white fish, 50muG per 100g.

Fair sources include:

- wholemeal bread, 20muG per 100g;
- white flour, 14muG per 100g;
- rice (uncooked weight), 10muG per 100g;
- bananas, 10muG per 100g;
- beef, 10muG per 100g;
- ham, 8muG per 100g;
- eggs, 8muG per 100g.

Poor sources are:

- chicken, lamb and pork, 3muG per 100g;
- fruits, 2–5muG per 100g;
- cow's milk, 0.2muG per 100g;
- human milk, 0.3muG per 100g (which is enough for a new baby).

The worst is goat's milk, which contains no folate at all.

One of the problems with folate is that it is easily destroyed by cooking or lost by soaking in water as it leaches into the water you throw away. On the plus side, vitamin C, found in fruit and vegetables, increases the absorption of folate, but it, too, is destroyed by cooking.

## How much folate does my body need?

Your body uses 100–200muG of folate every day – more if you are pregnant or ill. A normal Western diet provides 500–700mg daily, but only half of this is absorbed. Even so, you will build up a reserve of 10–15mg, which is enough to last you for three or four months, with normal usage, but is not enough to cover the extra demands of a pregnancy.

### Pushpa

Pushpa was already pregnant when she and Eddie came to Cornwall, leaving her big, close family behind in India. She was 22 and young for her age, because she had had a protected upbringing. She felt shy and strange in England: no one in the area spoke Gujerati and she was diffident about speaking English. That is why Pushpa didn't go to the antenatal clinic or get to know the doctor whose list she was on. She felt too exhausted to face the hassle and effort, and she could not have explained – in English – about her headaches, her tingling hands and her tongue feeling funny.

Her weight had stayed the same since she left India, despite the pregnancy. She did not feel like eating unfamiliar foods and, in the end, she ate very little apart from rice and some milk, which she thought would nourish the baby. (Milk is a poor supplier of folate, however, and she hardly ate any vitamin C-containing foods, which would have helped.)

Pushpa's mother-in-law was a forthright Lancashire woman. So, when she came down from Manchester to see her son and daughter-in-law, she took matters in hand immediately and with energy. Pushpa was marched off to the doctor's surgery where her mother-in-law explained Pushpa's symptoms for her, to start with. The tests showed that Pushpa had macrocytic anaemia of pregnancy because she was short of folate ('macrocytic' just means big cells). Apart from the extra demands the baby was making on her folate reserves, Pushpa's diet had been sadly lacking in this vitamin. She was soon being dragooned into eating what Eddie's mother called 'proper dinners' of meat and two vegetables. She also had to take folate tablets every day. Even so, little Shireen came ten days early.

Now, eight months later, the baby is thriving, Eddie is proud and Pushpa is well and much more confident. Her mother-in-law is in Manchester and the young couple are making new friends.

## Aplastic anaemia

This, fortunately, is rare as it is a very serious form of anaemia. It can affect people of any age, but the peak for suffering from it is around 30. Like many other forms of anaemia, it comes on insidiously. There is a progressive fall-off in the production of all the elements required for blood – red cells, white cells and platelets. Because of the lack of platelets (responsible for clotting), spontaneous bleeding is likely, with nosebleeds, blood in the urine and little spots of bleeding in the skin, lips and mouth. Also, bruises crop up anywhere. The sufferer is vulnerable to infections because the body's defences – the white blood cells – are drastically reduced.

## *What are the causes of aplastic anaemia?*

They are as follows:

- in half the cases the cause is never discovered: these are called 'idiopathic' illnesses, which means they derive from internal sources;
- congenital – something in the genes;
- a hypersensitivity to certain drugs that are perfectly harmless to other people, such as phenylbutazone (Butazolidin), sulphon-amides and gold preparations;
- it can follow on from viral hepatitis and some other illnesses caused by viruses;
- if there are toxins in the system, such as insecticides, benzene and so on;
- if there has been exposure to radiation.

None of these 'causes' operates by itself as most people don't react to them in this way. We do not yet know why the blood manufacturing process in the bone marrow is switched off in the unlucky ones.

## *What are the treatments for aplastic anaemia?*

### *Bone marrow transplant*

This needs to be taken from someone whose marrow is compatible with that of the ill person (usually a relative) as this gives the best chance of recovery for those under 50. It is especially likely to be effective in children.

### *Other treatments*

These include transfusions of red blood cells and platelets (the fluid part of the blood is not in short supply), antibiotics, to keep infections at bay, and certain steroids to stimulate the bone marrow.

*What is the outlook?*

There is no denying that this is a very dangerous illness. However, the small but real chance of spontaneous improvement and recovery makes it worth continuing with energetic treatment indefinitely.

*Billy*

Billy was $4\frac{1}{2}$ and due to start school in September. He was the youngest of three and seemed to pick up all the viruses the others brought home from school. In the last few months, he had been under the weather more often than not. All his liveliness – and mischief – had been siphoned off with the last bout of illness and, instead of improving, he was getting worse. He was coughing and snuffling non-stop and looked like a little ghost. Then the frightening nosebleeds began, and little haemorrhages appeared on his lips and in his mouth (little bleeds into and under the skin). He was admitted to the children's hospital and aplastic anaemia confirmed by the blood tests.

Blood transfusions kept Billy going for a short while, but it soon became clear that he was fighting a losing battle. Only a bone marrow transplant held out any hope. His mother's bone marrow turned out to be compatible, but there were many weeks of anxiety after the operation. Would the transplant be rejected? Billy hovered on the brink for what seemed a lifetime, but he did survive. Now it seems hard to believe that the nightmare of three years ago happened as Billy is a normal seven-year-old. He was one of the lucky ones.

# 9

# Anaemia due to damaged red cells

As we have seen, the red blood cells carry vital haemoglobin. If, for any reason the cells are broken, the haemoglobin leaks out and is lost – apart from the iron it contains, which is reabsorbed. In the normal course of events, your red blood cells wear out anyway when they are 110–120 days old, and are destroyed. Some large white cells called macrophages (the name means 'big biters') swallow them up. This takes place in the spleen, which is under your ribs on the left side of your body, and the liver, on the right, and a little in the bone marrow. The remains are disposed of, with the other waste, in the urine and the motions.

Excessive and premature destruction of the red cells is called haemolysis, which means blood melting, and there are several causes of this. Although the bone marrow will pull out all the stops to replace the red cells that have been lost, it may not be able to do it fast enough. The result is haemolytic anaemia. The spleen and liver are also having to work hard, to clear away the broken and discarded cells, and they may increase in size, like a muscle that is exercised more than usual. In some circumstances, the red cells start leaking before they reach the spleen and the haemoglobin spills straight into the bloodstream. One indication of this is haemoglobin appearing in the urine, which may look almost black, and excess blood pigment in the liver may form into gallstones. Also, the skin and the whites of the eyes are stained yellow, as well as, of course all the ordinary symptoms of anaemia – fatigue, pallor under the jaundice, shortness of breath, poor sleep, palpitations and so on.

## *What are the causes of haemolytic anaemia?*

These fall into two groups:

- acquired;
- hereditary.

## *Acquired haemolytic anaemia*

### *Autoimmune haemolytic disease*

To recap, autoimmune disorders are those in which the body's defences attack a group of its own cells – in this case, the red blood corpuscles. This can start up at any age and it is more likely if there are others in your family who have it or if any of you has one of the other autoimmune problems, for example diabetes or rheumatoid arthritis.

There are two kinds of autoimmune haemolytic disease: 'warm' and 'cold'. Most cases are of the warm type, and warm here means blood heat. It can come out of the blue or secondarily to ulcerative colitis, SLE (see page 65) or certain drugs. Methyldopa (Aldomet) is often involved.

The cold type, by contrast, is triggered by cold weather and is often associated with episodes of blood in the urine. It can also follow such infections as glandular fever and some varieties of pneumonia.

In both types, there will also be the usual symptoms of anaemia, and they can range from mild to severe, and there is likely to be noticeable jaundice. You may also develop an enlarged spleen or liver, but they do not hurt. In a bad case you may be feverish, vomit and feel absolutely knocked out. A diagnosis of these diseases would be confirmed by the results of a Coombs test, which would show the presence of antibodies on the red cells, and the blood film, which would show characteristically abnormal cells.

These diseases are treated with the steroid medicine prednisolone, but if that doesn't work and the symptoms are troublesome, the next option is surgical removal of the spleen. This is usually very effective, but you have to carry a card with you afterwards, to warn doctors who don't know you of the situation (see page 91).

### *Shortage of vitamin $B_{12}$ or folate*

Either of these shortages is likely to lead to poorly developed red blood cells that are too weak to last out their full lifespan. They are destroyed by the normal macrophage mechanism in the spleen, but too many are disposed of, too soon and so haemolytic anaemia is then added to the vitamin $B_{12}$ or folate deficiency anaemia.

## Fragmentation

This is a breaking up of the red cells. It can happen in someone who has an artificial heart valve as the cells catch on it as they pass through it. High blood pressure of the so-called malignant type (although this has nothing to do with cancer) or septicaemia (an infection in the bloodstream) can also damage the red cells so that the haemoglobin leaks out.

## Secondary effects of certain physical illnesses

Liver and kidney disorders, malaria and others can cause haemolytic anaemia as a side-effect.

## Other types of damage

Chemicals, poisonous snake or spider bites, severe burns, the drugs dapsone and salazopyrine, in people sensitive to them, can all cause haemolytic anaemia.

## Isoimmune haemolytic disease

There are two types:

- the result of an incompatible blood transfusion;
- haemolytic disease of the newborn.

An incompatible blood transfusion is a rarity, and due to human error, despite checks and counterchecks. Fortunately, the reaction is usually obvious as soon as the person receives the first small amount of the wrong blood, and the accident is likely to occur in hospital where appropriate treatment is at hand.

Haemolytic disease of the newborn arises when mother and baby have different blood groups and antibodies in the mother's blood attack the baby's red cells before it is born. The best-known reason for this is that the baby inherits the rhesus factor from its father, but the mother does not have the same factor in her blood. Tests for the rhesus factor are routinely made in early pregnancy for this reason. If the mother-to-be's blood is rhesus-negative – the less common type – the father's blood is tested also. If he is rhesus-positive, there is around a 1 in 20 chance that the baby will be at risk of its mother's blood reacting against its red cells. When this situation exists, the mother's serum is tested for antibodies around weeks 32 to 36 of the pregnancy and, in any event, arrangements are made for the birth to take place in hospital, where preventive measures and treatment as necessary can be applied.

An affected baby will be born with a big liver and spleen, and develop jaundice within a few hours of its birth. Because of the destruction of many of the baby's red corpuscles, it will be very anaemic. These problems will be treated by giving the baby blood transfusions for the anaemia and light therapy for the jaundice.

Commoner, but far less serious than the rhesus factor, is ABO incompatibility between mother and child. The ordinary blood groups are A, B, AB and O. If a group O mother is carrying an A, B or AB baby, it may be slightly anaemic and perhaps slightly jaundiced when it is born, but there is no need to worry about this.

## Andrew

He was not young any more – an old-looking 75, in fact. Andrew complained – with more accuracy than he realized – that his blood was thin. Because of his arthritis, he could only get around at a snail's pace, certainly never fast enough to warm himself up. And he had no comfortable padding of flesh and fat to help in this, although his wife gave him a cooked breakfast every morning, a midday dinner with meat and vegetables and an evening snack by the television.

Andrew's main complaint was of feeling cold. His fingers would go white and dead when everyone else felt perfectly warm. At best his feet and hands were blue, while in general his skin was the colour of parchment. Weary of her husband's moaning, Muriel made him go to the surgery. The doctor checked Andrew over and took some blood for a test.

The next week, the doctor explained that the results showed Andrew to be slightly anaemic, but not short of iron or vitamin $B_{12}$, so there was no point in taking supplements of these, which Muriel thought would be necessary. Andrew's anaemia was of the cold autoimmune haemolytic type, as abnormal-looking red cells were seen when his blood sample was looked at under the microscope.

There were two possible treatments: steroids or removal of the spleen, neither of which was very likely to help. A trial of

87

the steroids made Andrew feel worse, and he was not ill enough to warrant surgery at his age on the off-chance that this would benefit him. The answer – which Andrew approved of – was to turn up the thermostat on the central heating and wear a thermal vest, long johns and mittens indoors, bedsocks at night and thermal socks and gloves outside.

## Hereditary haemolytic anaemia

The trait that makes you prone to hereditary anaemia is, as you might expect, in your genes, and it may have had an effect even before you were born or else only show up years later. Sometimes it needs a special trigger to set off the symptoms or it may never bother you at all. The hereditary anaemias are of three types:

- those resulting from abnormal forms of haemoglobin, such as thalassaemia;
- those caused by an enzyme deficiency, which is when the body hasn't learned the trick of making one of the complicated chemicals necessary to control the metabolism;
- where the red blood cells have a weak 'skin'.

## Sickle cell disease and sickle cell anaemia

This is by far the most important of these kinds of anaemia. Although, as we saw earlier, it is commonplace all over Africa, parts of India, the Middle East and the Mediterranean countries, it is nowadays no longer a rarity in the West.

The key feature of the disease is a variation in the chemical structure of the person's haemoglobin, which makes the red blood cells prone to change shape. Interestingly, the sickle cell trait occurs if you have only one of the sickling genes, as opposed to the two that are associated with sickle cell anaemia itself. With the trait only, less than half of your haemoglobin will be of the abnormal type. Thus, the only effect this will have on you is that, as you get older, your kidneys will not be able make really concentrated orangey-yellow urine – unless, that is, you are in a situation where you are relatively short of oxygen, as happens when you are at high altitudes, as we saw with Francesca, page 7. A long surgical operation under a general anaesthetic can have a similar effect and set off a sickling crisis, which is when the red cells change from discs to a sickle or new moon shape. When the cells are this odd shape, they can get caught up and block a blood vessel, causing acute pain, often in the abdomen or a bone.

If you inherit the sickling gene from both your parents, a large proportion of your red cells will contain the abnormal haemoglobin and will be sickle-shaped. These cells do not survive as well as normal cells and you will develop a long-term form of haemolytic anaemia, punctuated by the typical crises.

This anaemia, like any other, makes you feel generally tired out, unable to play sport or take other vigorous exercise for more than a brief stint, and be extra susceptible to infection. For instance, if you knock or cut yourself, healing may be slow. Of course, you may have any of the other general symptoms of anaemia, such as headaches, palpitations, poor sleep and so on.

The crises are of two types:

- those in which there is a sudden wave of increased red cell destruction, so that the haemoglobin level falls dramatically;
- the blockage, or infarction, variety, when the cells become jammed in a blood vessel.

In babies this often affects the fingers and toes, perhaps because the vessels are so tiny that they are easily blocked. Either kind of crisis may be triggered by an infection, becoming chilled or dehydrated or there being a lack of oxygen, but it passes in a few days. In the second, painful type, the victim will need powerful painkillers to tide them over the worst, and in the blood loss type, a transfusion of concentrated red corpuscles. Antibiotics will also be required to deal with, or ward off, any infection.

Life isn't all crisis and drama, however, even if you do have sickle cell anaemia. Some people may go through life being only mildly anaemic and subject to what they believe are rheumatic pains from time to time without anyone realizing the underlying cause until a blood test is done for a quite unconnected reason.

*The thalassaemias – alpha and beta, major and minor*

These, like sickle cell disease, are due to a quirk in the chemistry of the haemoglobin, and they are most frequently found in the same areas, plus a huge swathe of South-East Asia.

Beta thalassaemia minor occurs when only one of your parents hands down the gene. It involves a mild anaemia without either iron or vitamin deficiency. Instead, the anaemia derives from an increased loss of red cells as a result of their faulty haemoglobin. Because of the extra blood-manufacturing activity necessary to replace the lost cells and their haemoglobin, supplements of folate may be necessary. There is not usually a shortage of vitamin $B_{12}$ nor iron as this is recycled when the red cells are destroyed.

Beta thalassaemia major occurs when both parents supply the relevant genes to their child and, sadly, the result is tragic. Even transfusions cannot help a child with these genes to survive.

Alpha thalassaemia is caused by different genes from the ones involved in the beta varieties, but the effects of the minor and major forms are similar. The minor form produces a type of anaemia that is problematical, but the major form is a disaster.

## G6PD deficiency

Glucose-6-phosphate dehydrogenase is an enzyme that protects the red blood cells from the damaging effects of certain medicines. The deficiency affects males only, but women can be the carriers of the faulty gene, so it is a gender-linked disorder.

If you have inherited a lack of G6PD, your red cells may be devastated by such common medicines as aspirin, sulphonamides or antimalarials, among others, and also by the broad, or fava, bean. The reaction – haemolysis of your red cells – starts within a few days of ingesting the medicine or beans. You become anaemic from loss of blood, with jaundice and, in some long-term cases, gallstones. It is vital to track down what is causing the problem and stop taking it as then the illness will subside. In future you will need to avoid the drugs that commonly cause this problem for those with this deficiency and try any new one cautiously.

## Hereditary spherocytosis

In this disorder, the membrane, or skin, of the red blood cells does not develop properly and so the cells cannot hold their special disc shape with concave sides. Instead, they become round, like balls. They then easily break, spilling their haemoglobin, and are destroyed in the spleen, leaving the person short of red cells and, thus, anaemic.

The illness may be mild and hardly noticeable or very severe, depending on the numbers of red cells involved. The spleen is usually enlarged because of the extra work it has to do. Jaundice comes and goes, depending on how many red cells are destroyed, and gallstones, made from blood pigment, may cause attacks of acute pain in the upper abdomen. Leg ulcers, because of poor healing after trivial injuries, are also quite common in those with this disease and there may be episodes when there is a sudden, rapid loss of red cells, with a sharp worsening of the other symptoms of anaemia, such as chest pain, dimming of vision, breathlessness, throbbing in the ears or head, tingling hands and so on. If haemolytic episodes like this, or attacks of pain from gallstones threaten the sufferer's normal lifestyle and activities, the surgical removal of the spleen usually produces a striking and permanent change for the better. After this operation, the patient must always carry a splenectomy card, to inform any doctor who may treat them that they are unduly susceptible to major infections, and to one bug in particular – the pneumococcus of pneumonia.

*Ron*

Ron was 40 and, as far as he was concerned, there was absolutely nothing wrong with him – that is, until he went out to lunch that Sunday.

An aunt of his wife's had invited them – their only wealthy relative. She was known to be slightly eccentric and very touchy, so Ron was on his best behaviour. Aunt Sybil had cooked them a meal of lamb and bean stew, using broad beans from her garden. Ron didn't much care for the meal, but, to be polite, he allowed himself to be persuaded to have a second, huge helping. It was such a pleasure to feed someone who appreciated good, plain, English cooking, purred Aunt Sybil.

The reaction came a few days later. Ron felt like death and looked it: ashy pale with a tinge of yellow. His urine was dark with blood and he felt sick and dizzy. His head throbbed.

Ron's doctor sent him to hospital, where a number of

screening tests identified the cause of his haemolytic anaemia as G6PD deficiency.

Ron recovered in a week, although he looked washed out for a month or so longer while his lost blood was being restored by his bone marrow. Now he knows that he can't touch broad beans or take certain medicines, and he should start with small doses only of any new medicine to test its effect on him gently.

Ron's mother must have passed the G6PD gene to him. He wondered about her family: they had come from Canada. There are millions of people worldwide with G6PD deficiency, but it is most prevalent in the black population of the United States, and among the races subject to sickle cell disease.

# 10

## How to avoid becoming anaemic

Keeping healthy is not usually considered much fun by most people – tedious and tiring exercises, freezing cold fresh air, coating your skin with sunscreen when it is lovely and warm outside and remembering your posture when your instinct is to slump. However, the delightful news about the steps you should take to avoid anaemia is that they are enjoyable. They involve eating enough good food to ensure that you have plenty of the healthy blood-forming nutrients. This is the opposite of the usual wearisome diet routine – for women, at least – of feeling guilty about eating almost anything. As we may only absorb as little as 10 per cent of what we eat, we need to have enough, and to spare, of the vital ingredients, which are protein, iron and the vitamins $B_{12}$, C and folate. Calcium is useful, too, as it helps in the absorption of iron.

### *Protein*

As the globin of haemoglobin is itself a protein, this is a must. Proteins are composed of various amino acids. There are 20 of these, of which 8 are necessary for making human blood. Meat especially, but also the other foods from animal sources, such as milk, provide all the amino acids you need, as well as another essential, vitamin $B_{12}$. A mix of wholemeal bread and beans, in the ratio of 2 to 1, provides a little of each of the vital amino acids, but none of the vitamin $B_{12}$. And, of course, as the plant-based mixture is only 13 per cent protein, you would have to eat a huge amount of it to supply all you need.

Vegetarian foods that contain some protein are:

- soya, peas, beans and nuts – these provide the most;
- brown bread, brown rice and sweetcorn – these provide some;
- bananas and potatoes – but they hardly rate a mention.

An average adult in Britain eats around 65g ($2\frac{1}{2}$oz) of protein daily.

The absolute minimum is 40g (1½oz), and that must be of the first-class kind, which is meat, fish, poultry, eggs or hard cheese. It works out at about 10 per cent of your total intake. Children, mothers-to-be, those breastfeeding and men doing exceptionally heavy work need proportionately more – maybe even double. We also all need extra to help the body repair itself after loss of blood, whatever the cause, or an illness, an injury or a burn. Babies, of course, get their protein, and everything else, from milk, but it is not concentrated enough for older people (you would have to drink large quantities of it to satisfy your needs). Because of the importance of blood, the requirements of the bone marrow, where blood is produced, have priority over other parts when the available protein is sent around the body. If the supplies are meagre, your muscles and other organs may have to go short.

Those at risk of taking in too little protein are vegetarians, Asian people who rely mainly on chapattis and vegetables or rice, and those who need extra quantities of protein, mentioned above. They all need to include more meat, poultry, fish, eggs, cheese and milk in their diet.

## Iron

This is vital in making the other half of haemoglobin – the haem part. Iron is the constituent of blood that you are most liable to run short of. You can get it from:

- liver, corned beef, fresh beef and lamb, old-fashioned treacle and oatmeal – these are the best sources of iron in the diet;
- eggs, dark chocolate, peas, beans, Allbran and bread – the next best sources;
- fish, milk, nuts, fruit and root vegetables – the least useful sources of iron.

Spinach – perhaps thanks to Popeye – has a great reputation for being a provider of iron, and, indeed, it does contain more iron than other vegetables. However, unfortunately, you need about four times a normal size helping to do much good, and the same goes for broccoli, cabbage and Brussels sprouts. In any case, a normal mixed diet that includes meat gives you more iron than any vegetarian one, and also enables you to absorb it better. Calcium – from all kinds of dairy products – also helps you to absorb the iron, as does vitamin C (found in fresh fruit) while tea and the phytic acid in unmilled cereals inhibit it.

The groups of people requiring extra iron are the same as those needing extra supplies of protein, but, in addition, all women who have periods have a 5 per cent deficit that they need to make up throughout each year.

## *Vitamin B$_{12}$ and folate*

These two vitamins function together in the making of blood. Vitamin B$_{12}$ comes solely from animal sources and folate from plants and some animal products, while fruit and vegetables, bread and cereals do not provide us with any vitamin B$_{12}$. Fresh green vegetables, especially spinach and broccoli, and liver contain the most folate. Wholemeal bread, bananas, beef, ham and eggs are the next best providers of folate, but fruit, milk, lamb, pork and poultry don't supply us with any.

The body has a big reserve of vitamin B$_{12}$ as a contingency measure, so you don't need to eat vitamin B$_{12}$-rich foods every day. With folate, however, you keep only enough to last for a few weeks, so it is wise to keep this store topped up. Again, those who are still growing, including, by proxy, women who are pregnant, and the other groups mentioned above have the greatest need for adequate supplies of these vitamins.

## *Vitamin C*

There is no excuse for anyone to run low in this vitamin as it abounds in foods that are a treat to eat, such as:

- strawberries, raspberries, blackcurrants and cherries in season, and all the year round from overseas; citrus fruits, mangoes and pineapple are excellent sources;
- salads and raw green vegetables, tomatoes and peppers are also first-class sources of vitamin C;

- apples, plums, pears and melons are not such good sources, but are still useful;
- milk and meat supply us with none.

## How to get the most benefit from your food

- Unnecessary cooking wipes out most of the vitamin C and folate in your food as they are destroyed by heat. Raw is best, and lightly cooked better than well-cooked. Chips are better, vitamin-wise, than boiled or roast potatoes as the cooking time is shorter.
- Steam rather than boil your vegetables, because both iron and vitamins are lost in the water.
- Oatmeal, wholegrain wheat and cereals contain iron, but they are also full of phytic acid and this prevents the absorption of both iron and another useful mineral, calcium. Tea also inhibits the absorption of iron, so don't drink too much of it and don't make it too strong. Coffee, though, does not have this effect, so you could drink coffee instead – still in moderate quantites, of course!
- Don't take your iron pills with or after food: they are absorbed better if they are taken before a meal.
- Take iron tablets at reasonable intervals as up to six hours after each dose, your body won't take in any more iron.
- Don't keep your fruit and vegetables out in the open or peel or chop them some time before you are going to eat them as exposure to the air means a loss of vitamin C.
- It is unwise to be a vegan: at least take some cheese, eggs and milk, and fish, too, if possible.

## Watch your alcohol intake

Alcohol is one of the pleasures in life that you need not miss out on, but, like gambling, it can be harmful if you have too much – especially if your taste runs to spirits. Substantial drinking on a regular basis can lead you into anaemia by several routes:

- a direct poisoning effect of the alcohol on your red blood cells and also the bone marrow – the red cells become oversized – even before you are anaemic;

- a strain is put on the liver as it has to deal with all the alcohol, so it cannot fulfil its role properly in the metabolism of your blood;
- inflammation of the digestive tract (think of the feeling of warmth as a mouthful of whisky or vodka goes down) leading to little, unnoticed haemorrhages and, in the later stages, some big ones – either way it means a loss of blood and anaemia;
- folate deficiency because of an impaired metabolism;
- a generally poor diet as you may use a drink as a pick-you-up when you really need a proper meal, and you may lose your appetite – many drinkers can't face any breakfast;
- alcoholic gastritis may interfere with the production of the intrinsic factor in the stomach and lead to pernicious anaemia.

## *Could you be losing blood without realizing?*

The leaking or seeping away of a teaspoonful of blood per day is enough to make you anaemic, and unnoticed blood loss is a very common cause of anaemia. If you have any of the symptoms of anaemia, consider if bleeding from any of these areas could be responsible for it:

- piles;
- hiatus hernia;
- peptic ulcer;
- diverticular disease (age changes in the colon);
- ulcerative colitis;
- long, frequent or heavy periods;
- other gynaecological problems;
- nosebleeds as a result of infection or high blood pressure.

## *Think about your family*

Do you have any relatives who have anaemia? Is there any tendency in the family to have autoimmune disorders? These include diabetes, vitiligo (see page 64), rheumatoid arthritis, lupus, thyroid disorders, pernicious anaemia, autoimmune gastritis, dermatomyositis, certain liver disorders and Goodpasture's kidney disease.

If you or a relative has any of these problems, this makes you more vulnerable to anaemia. You should then be extra vigilant for the early, vague symptoms of anaemia and – if you are in doubt – have your blood tested.

## *Medicines that may trigger anaemia*

Although usually the following medicines do not have anaemia as a side-effect, this can occur:

- painkillers, such as aspirin, phenacetin and the non-steroidal anti-inflammatory drugs (NSAIDs), such as ibuprofen (Brufen) used in the treatment of joint and rheumatic pain;
- steroids, such as prednisolone;
- gold, phenylbutazone (Butazolidin), isoniazid;
- phenytoin (Epanutin), primidone, phenobarbitone, sodium valproate;
- oral contraceptives;
- neomycin, metformin (Glucophage);
- penicillins, tetracycline, nitrofurantoin (Furadantin), sulphonamides;
- carbimazole;
- captopril, nifedipine (taken for high blood pressure);
- mood-altering drugs, such as amitriptyline (Tryptizol), chlorpromazine, mianserin, clozapine, dothiepin;
- quinidine, chlorpropamide;
- Tagamet, Zantac;
- dapsone, salazopyrine.

## *If you are over 70, read this*

If you are 70 or more, you are special: the ordinary rules don't apply. Your body, to make things easy for you, is adjusting to suit a less active lifestyle. You still want to feel fully fit, but you won't be aiming to beat Tim Henman at tennis or out-kick Gazza on the football field. It is only sensible to scale down on the athletic front and concentrate on the areas where your interests now lie.

Your body will shift gear into a more economical mode, so play along with it to achieve the maximum benefit. For example, why should your body waste resources on producing pigment for your hair when it looks just as elegant white or grey? For women, it would be crazy for the body to go on and on pouring out hormones in an endless rhythm of blood-wasting periods on the off-chance of your wanting a baby now. For men and women there is no call, at this stage, for you to carry a heavy skeleton and powerful muscles when lighter equipment will serve the purpose adequately.

On the other hand, your heart isn't fazed by your age and, barring accidents, it will go on beating steadily until you are 90 or more. However, it may take a moment or two longer than it used to for your circulation to adjust when you get up from a low chair, and although your lungs will easily take in all the oxygen you need for ordinary living, you will probably find that it takes a little more effort to sing or make a speech.

## *Your blood*

This is affected by the normal changes in your digestive system. Your stomach will be making slightly less acid than it used to and this means that some substances are less well absorbed. These include some of the essentials for making blood, namely iron and vitamins $B_{12}$ and C. At the same time, you may produce a little less intrinsic factor. These changes mean that you must make sure that you eat an orange daily or have the equivalent in tablet form to supply your need for vitamin C, together with meat – preferably red – two or three times a week for its vitamin $B_{12}$, and other protein foods as well. These are cheese, fish, chicken, bacon and eggs. Lentils and other beans provide some protein, too, but nuts are too difficult to digest. Remember, you need almost as much protein at 75 as you did at 35, as well as vegetables for their folate content.

Getting enough iron is a common problem. In fact, up to 20 per cent of those over 70 have iron deficiency anaemia and so feel tired unnecessarily. The reduction in stomach acid is one causative factor, but the other is down to you. Because your teeth may not be as efficient as they were when you were younger, it is often less trouble to eat a bun or a biscuit than to cut up some fruit to eat. However, you need the vitamin C in the fruit to help you absorb sufficient iron from your food. Dairy products, too, help the absorption of iron, because of the calcium in them.

Foods that supply iron include meat, liver, Allbran, plain chocolate and oatmeal. Porridge, too, is an excellent provider of iron, but you must take milk with it, to neutralize the phytic acid.

You may feel that now you don't need such big meals as you did when you were younger, but make sure that you don't also cut down on the nutrients you need for your blood. You can safely reduce your intake of fillers, such as biscuits, cakes, potatoes, rice, bread and pasta, but keep to good portions of the foods mentioned above.

### Warning signs that you may be becoming anaemic

These are:

- weakness and weariness;
- you are unsteady when you walk;
- forgetfulness or muddled thinking;
- loss of sensation or pins and needles in your feet and hands;
- a sore tongue.

If you experience one or more of the above, see your doctor.

### Symptoms that are normal

Something *not* to worry about are those red, then purple and brownish spots on the skin of your hands and forearms – those areas subject to mild daily wear and tear. If you are over 60, they are harmless reminders of maturity. There is a loss of the elastic tissue in the walls of your smallest blood vessels, allowing a little leakage, and the macrophages (the cells that clear away old or broken red blood cells) are not as quick off the mark as they were when you were 21, so these tiny haemorrhages take a long time to disappear.

Another normal change is for you to have a lower level of haemoglobin in your blood as it goes down a little from the age of 60, and more sharply at 70 because you then have a less demanding metabolism. Anything over 10g/dl is perfectly acceptable at 70 or over and does not spell anaemia.

# *What is a sensible diet?*

The figures given in Table 10.1 are a guide to the intakes required by different age groups and sexes, but to allow for the inevitable wastage, you will always need to consume more than these bare calorific requirements.

Table 10.1   The amounts of calories you need

| Sector of the population | Age group | Number of calories (daily) |
|---|---|---|
| Both sexes | 0–1 year | 800 |
| | 2–3 | 1400 |
| | 5–7 | 1800 |
| Boys | 9–12 | 2500 |
| | 15–18 | 3000 |
| Girls | 9–12 | 2300 |
| | 15–18 | 2300 |
| Men | 18–35 | 2700–3600 |
| | 60+ | 1900 |
| Women | 18–35 | 2200 |
| during pregnancy | | 2400 |
| | 60+ | 1700 |

## *Some suggestions for anti-anaemia meals*
Of course you can add fillers or seconds of the following according to your appetite and personal needs.

### *Breakfasts*
- Porridge or muesli with honey and milk, orange juice, toast and so on, coffee or tea.
- Grilled tomatoes or mushrooms or baked beans on wholemeal toast, and coffee or tea.
- Boiled, poached or scrambled egg with toast and spread and an orange or other fruit, plus a drink.
- Ham or bacon with tomatoes and toast, plus coffee or tea or fruit juice.
- Three fruits, crispbread and soft cheese and coffee, tea or fruit juice.

101

*Lunches*

- Sandwich or soft roll (wholemeal if possible) filled with cheese and pickle, ham or beef and mustard or chicken and mayonnaise, with a tomato or fruit, plus a yogurt, coffee, hot chocolate, fruit juice, cider or beer.
- A jacket potato with a filling of meat, cheese, ham, tuna, chicken and peppers, egg, coleslaw or baked beans, with a piece of fruit or salad and a drink.
- Meat, ham, egg or cheese with salad and a brown roll, plus a yogurt or a piece of apple pie and a drink.

*Suppers*

- A glass of wine – optional.
- 120g ($4\frac{1}{2}$oz) of lean meat, or the equivalent, with a salad of raw or steamed vegetables – as much variety as possible – with a dairy product in the second course, such as yogurt, custard or cheese.

*Main courses*

- Braised liver, leeks and potatoes.
- Bean and other vegetable curry and brown rice.
- Lamb chop, broccoli, carrots and potatoes.
- Slice of steak, onions, mushrooms and tomatoes and a roll or some sliced bread.
- Stir-fried chicken and mixed vegetables and naan bread.
- White fish, spinach and chips.
- Roast or casseroled beef or lamb, with green vegetables and potatoes.
- Omelette, peppers and tomatoes with a roll or sliced bread.

*Desserts*

- Baked apple with sultanas and ice-cream.
- Fruit pie.
- Egg custard and stewed fruit.
- Grilled grapefruit and a chocolate biscuit.
- Cheese with an apple or crackers.
- Fruit sorbet, biscuit.
- Raspberry mousse.

- Baked banana
- And, of course, fresh fruit at any time.

### *Note for babies and young children*

Babies must start mixed feeding by the time they are four months old, with purées of vegetables and fruits, then a month or so later, purées with some meat incorporated. From eight months, minced food is manageable, and, from a year old onwards, eggs are very useful. Fruit juice should replace milk as the drink to take *with* meals, starting from six months.

It is necessary to introduce vegetable purées early because from around three to four months your baby may start to run short of iron: even the very best breast or other milk does not supply enough. Also babies adapt to solids more easily if they start to be given them from four months rather than later.

From the toddler stage onwards, your child can digest most of the foods you have at home, but is still liable to choke on hard bits and lumps until the age of $2\frac{1}{2}$ to 3.

It is in childhood that healthy eating habits are learned – ones that will last a lifetime. As an adult, you are responsible for working out your own good habits.

Bon appetit!

# Index